Essential Supplements for Women

Essential Supplements for Women

What Every Woman Should Know About Vitamins, Minerals, Enzymes, & Amino Acids

Carolyn Reuben, C.A.,
& Joan Priestley, M.D.

A Perigee Book

Perigee Books are published by
The Putnam Publishing Group
200 Madison Avenue
New York, NY 10016

This book is intended to serve as a general reference source of dietary supplements for women. The reader is advised to consult with a physician in planning a proper regimen of diet and exercise to meet the reader's individual needs. The author and the publisher expressly disclaim responsibility for any adverse effects or unforeseen consequences resulting from the use of any information contained herein.

LIBRARY OF CONGRESS CATALOGING-IN-PUBLICATION DATA

Reuben, Carolyn, date.
  Essential supplements for women: what every woman should know
about vitamins, minerals, enzymes, and amino acids / Carolyn Reuben
and Joan Priestley.
       p.   cm.
  Bibliography: p.
  Includes index.
  ISBN 0-399-51437-6
  1. Women—Diseases—Popular works.   2. Women—Diseases—
Nutritional aspects.   3. Dietary supplements.   I. Priestley, Joan,
date. II. Title.
RG121.R48   1988   88-1571 CIP
618.1'0654—dc19

Printed in the United States of America
1 2 3 4 5 6 7 8 9 10

Acknowledgments

Carolyn thanks: Dominick Bosco, for giving me the chance to write this book; Adrienne Ingrum, our editor, for the original idea, for choosing us, and for translating the manuscript into a book; Robert Schuster, our agent, for manifesting the contract; the following executive officers, who allowed me free rein in their company libraries: William Thompson, chairman of the board, and John Foster, technical director, for the William T. Thompson Company; Jeff Katke, president of Metagenics; Marjorie and Don Tyson of Tyson and Associates; and Kenneth Rosenberg, chief operating officer of Pharmavite Corporation. And Ron Martin, manager of technical services for the William T. Thompson Company, whose assistance was crucial to the research for this book; and Paul Bolar, director of quality assurance and regulatory affairs for Pharmavite, who found needed references; Deanna Nipp, reference librarian at Rutgers University Science and Medicine Library, who took books home to search for references for me; William Lamers, M.D., and Elizabeth Lamers, for sending clippings to a needy stranger; Patti Wolff, D.C.; Janet Zand, O.M.D.; James Privitera, M.D.; Larry Eckstein, M.D.; Valentine Birds, M.D.; Virginia Flanagan, M.D.; David Katzin, M.D.; Murray Susser, M.D.; and William C. Douglass, M.D., for their insights and personal stories of nutritional treatments; Melvyn Werbach, M.D.; Jeffrey Bland, Ph.D.; Jonathan Wright, M.D.; Alan Gaby, M.D.; and the late Alan Nittler, M.D., for their inspiration and practical information in the field of medical nutrition; Eytan ben Sheviya, for introducing me to health consciousness; Ernestine Rita Salter, my grandmother, who isn't here to share in the *nachas* of my first book, but who always insisted I should forget all my other *mishegas* and stick to writing; Carol Noonan, Judy and Shimon Lipkin, Leni Wander, and Tozienka Rubin for financial and emotional support as deep and as dear as friendship goes; Stacey Konkoff, Tia Hoffer, Mildred Walter, Alesia Barbour, and Ninette D'Alessandro for helping me stay organized; Moonyene Lew for her postpartum soup recipe; Jonathan Reich, for teaching me to use my computer, helping me get the manuscript in on time, supporting me in so many ways, and blessing me with the child of my dreams; Natanya, my gift from the universe, for forcing me to balance writing and research with nurturance and play; Marcia Schmiegelow, Johanna Rhoads, and the late Carolyn Leeper, for my peace of mind (and the peaceful hours alone in my home/office) while Natanya was under their care the nine months it took to birth this book.

To Betty Sylvia Reuben and Jack Reuben, who live their love of truth and justice, respect for humankind, and joy in learning, who always encouraged me and supported me both financially and emotionally through all my enthusiasms and adventures, and who model in their personal lives the values that are the basis for true health, not only of individuals, but of our social body as well.

—C.R.

To the many wonderful and courageous doctors and patients who took the time and interest to educate me about the politics and practice of nutritional medicine, with special thanks to Jeffrey Bland, Ph.D., my major hero and mentor, and a prince for our time.

—J.P.

Contents

Supplements in the Woman's Body and Life-style

Women use nutritional supplements for many good reasons, such as to prevent the common cold, to prevent fragile bones, to have a healthy pregnancy and birth, or to have more energy and experience less fatigue or depression.

Whatever your particular reason, you join approximately 41 percent of all Americans and about 33 percent of all Canadians if you regularly consume vitamins and minerals. Food supplements are a multibillion dollar industry.

In spite of the medical profession's disapproval, individuals within that profession participate in this growing practice at a rate at times ahead of the rest of the population: In Washington State, 60 percent of dietitians surveyed in 1984 admitted to taking nutritional supplements, and in the 1982 data collection of an ongoing longitudinal study of 120,000 American nurses, 34 to 38 percent claimed to use a multivitamin regularly.

In fact, heretofore undiagnosed marginal deficiencies of vitamins and minerals are being recognized as the cause of a wide variety of vague complaints that bring women into physicians' offices: irritability, fatigue, difficulty concentrating, insomnia, muscle aches, tooth and gum problems, menstrual difficulties, and many other discomforts.

Before we plunge into the conditions that warrant life-style changes and the consumption of supplements, we want to present some facts about these controversial little packets of nutrients as well as our position on their use.

What's in a Vitamin?

"We build vitamins like Detroit builds cars," one vitamin company executive explained to us. "They don't manufacture their own glass, plastics, or metals. They assemble these materials into a car of their own design." So, too, vitamin distributors obtain their ingredients from major pharmaceutical concerns and then formulate their own combinations of these ingredients with their unique choice of excipients (inert substances that bind ingredients, make the tablet denser, and ease movement of ingredients through machinery).

Thus, Hoffmann-La Roche, manufacturer of the tranquilizer Valium, provides American vitamin distributors with vitamins A, C, E, and B complex. Eastman Kodak Company also produces a large portion of the nation's vitamin E. The Merck Company, the producer of the tranquilizer Elavil, and the A. E. Staley Manufacturing Company are other major sources of B vitamins.

Beware of advertising puffery when you read claims regarding "natural" sources of vitamin C such as acerola berries or rosehips. All the manufacturers have done is add a whisper of these substances to the ascorbic acid crystals they purchased from Hoffmann-La Roche.

Amino Acids

There are four grades of amino acids, ranging from the low "animal grade," suitable for cows, to the high "pharmaceutical grade," suitable for direct intravenous injection into humans. Prices vary accordingly. The higher the grade, the less possibility there is of contamination, so with amino acids, it's best to pay more and obtain the highest quality possible.

Natural vs. Synthetic

When chemists broke down many nutrients into their most elemental structure, they noticed that polarized light rotated through the molecules either to the left (called levo-rotary, from the Latin *laevus* meaning left, and abbreviated "l-") or to the right (called dextro-rotary, from the Latin *dexter* meaning right, and abbreviated "d-"). The abbreviation "dl-" means that part of the substance is rotating to the right and part to the left.

No one knows for sure whether direction of rotation has biological significance. Take the case of vitamin E. If the "natural" advocates are correct, our bodies can only use the fraction of E that rotates as nature created it, which is to the right, and so you actually are only using 100 I.U. of vitamin E for every 200 I.U. of dl-alpha tocopherol that you buy. However, a Canadian family of physicians, the Shutes, obtained good results using dl-alpha tocopherol in their pioneering treatment of heart conditions, so we aren't convinced either way. We suggest that you purchase the cheapest vitamin E available, probably dl-alpha tocopherol, and see if that works for you. After a few months, try d-alpha tocopherol, and compare your results. Your own body is the ultimate judge of effectiveness.

Minerals

Minerals like calcium, zinc, and iron have a positive electrical charge, as does the lining of your small intestine, where most nutrients are absorbed. Like charges repel each other, so to move minerals across the intestinal barrier and into the bloodstream, where they are used, it is necessary to negate the positive charge by binding it to a negatively charged molecule. When the negatively charged molecule is an amino acid, the compound is called a chelate. Minerals bound to amino acids are called chelated minerals and are the most easily absorbed.

Calcium: A Special Case

Media coverage of osteoporosis, the weakening of bones that often occurs as people age, has caused calcium consumption to shoot up in recent years. But some forms of calcium are less useful than others.

We think a chelated form is best for most people. Elderly women, however, may be deficient in stomach acid (hydrochloric acid), and chelated calcium needs an acidic environment for most efficient absorption. Consequently, elderly women may want to use calcium lactate or calcium gluconate, since neither of these compounds needs an acidic environment to be absorbed. The best choice for vegetarians is calcium citrate, which doesn't rely on animal products, and is adequately absorbed even by the elderly. We suggest that everyone avoid oyster shell calcium: It sounds natural and is definitely inexpensive, but it is made of the same calcium carbonate that composes an antacid pill. The last thing you want to eliminate is acid when taking calcium. In fact, people who take too many antacids over time can develop "milk alkali syndrome," in which unabsorbed calcium precipitates out of the blood and into joints and can cause eye and kidney damage as well. Calcium carbonate is also the most tightly bound of all the calcium forms and is, therefore, the most difficult to absorb even when acid is plentiful.

What's Inside?

If you want only absolutely natural ingredients, you won't take supplements at all, but will stick exclusively to food. Anything you buy in a bottle has been manipulated somehow. In fact, the vitamin D a vitamin distributor purchases from a pharmaceutical giant and carefully combines in its own preservative-free formula—slapping a big "natural" on the label—may already contain cottonseed oil, sugar, gelatin, modified food starch, methyl paraben, propyl paraben, potassium sorbate, BHT (butylated hydroxytoluene), and BHA (butylated hydroxyanisole) when it arrives at the distributor's door. The only way to find out what is really in a product is to request this information from the manufacturer.

As you try to figure out what is *really* in a supplement, also be aware that some suspicious-sounding substances are actually derived from natural sources and are benign, while some innocuous names hide ingredients that we recommend you avoid. Harmless excipients include silica (a mineral that blends ingredients); cellulose (plant fiber used as a filler); potassium alginate (a seaweed-based binder); and stearic acid, magnesium stearate, or calcium stearate (fatty acids that help move ingredients through tableting machinery).

Excipients to avoid include PVP (polyvinylpropylone povidone is a blood plasma extender used during World War II that may pass benignly through the body, or may attach to some nutrients and reduce the supplement's potency); any ingredient with the suffix "-ose" or "-ol" (ingredients with these suffixes, such as sucrose, mannose, and xylitol, are sweeteners); shellac coatings (which harden and can make intestinal absorption impossible—watch for undigested tablets in your stools, or contact the manufacturer and ask what coating they use); coloring agents (most contain sugar and chemicals, which make the liver work harder and force it to waste vitamin C and other nutrients to get rid of those chemicals); and gelatin capsules (of concern only to vegetarians, since the capsules are made from animal products).

Are They Working?

Ask your own body to reveal whether your supplement program is working. Do your symptoms return when you stop taking your supplements? Do they go away again once you restart your program? Do you feel nauseated or suffer stomach pain after taking your supplements? You must know why you are taking each supplement, if you are to recognize whether it is doing its job. If you have been ill for a long time, or have multiple problems, we can't emphasize enough the importance of seeing a nutrition-minded health-care provider for advice.

When to Take What

Zinc and iron tend to cause stomach distress, so take them with meals. Calcium is "nature's sleeping pill," so take it at night. And since amino acids are best absorbed on an empty stomach, take them between meals.

Caring for Supplements

The purer the original product, the longer it will remain potent. Even preservatives, however, won't keep a vitamin viable forever. The expiration date indicates when the product has only 90 percent of its original potency, unless otherwise specified on the label. Even without a printed date, don't use a bottle of vitamin A if it's more than one year old. Vitamin C and the B complex can be used somewhat longer. If you aren't sure of the product's age, the manufacturer can tell you if you provide the product lot number printed on the label.

Refrigeration protects oil-based supplements such as A and E from deterioration. Keep all supplements tightly closed, to protect them from moisture. And never store supplements in the glove compartment of the car, where they will be unprotected from heat.

Too Much of a Good Thing

Two young men who were identical twins took the incredible dose of 300,000 international units of vitamin A—the U.S. recommended dietary allowance, or RDA, for men is 5,000 I.U.—but only one developed symptoms of toxicity. Biochemical individuality is one reason why one individual is poisoned and another isn't by the same dose of a drug or vitamin, but that isn't the whole story. As one nutritional physician likes to tell patients, "It's not just your genes, it's also how you wear them." In fact, even in one person, "excess" doses of supplements vary from day to day. See for yourself how much vitamin C you can tolerate without developing diarrhea when you're ill, compared to when you are well.

It is not wise to assume that everything natural is safe. The water-soluble vitamins, B complex and C, move through the blood and into the fluid between cells. When you urinate, some of these vitamins are excreted. Although these vitamins aren't retained for long, massive doses over time can cause overload symptoms. The fat-soluble vitamins, A, D, and E, are stored wherever fat accumulates, such as in the liver, muscles, and skin. Extended excessive doses can cause quantities toxic to the individual to accumulate and symptoms of vitamin poisoning will result. Excess vitamin A during pregnancy can cause birth defects or miscarriage.

Overdoses necessitating medical intervention do not occur overnight but develop when an individual has ignored weeks or months of warning signs such as dry skin, severe headaches, hair loss, stiff joints, or tingling extremities. These conditions frequently reverse themselves when the offending supplement is discontinued.

The Politics of Caution

National health organizations used to harp on one point: Americans could obtain all their nutrients from a well-balanced diet. But study after study has revealed how imbalanced the American diet is. To cite only one example: A 1982 Department of Agriculture survey revealed that only 3 percent of Americans ate the recommended number of servings from the "four basic food groups." Where's the balance, when french fried potatoes frequently represent the category of vegetables for some misguided folks?

Combine ignorance with both biochemical individuality (including a possible ten fold variation in different individuals' vitamin needs) and the many "vitamin robbers" that threaten us on a daily basis, and you have a veritable chorus of causes for widespread malnourishment. Those everyday nutrient thieves include emotional stress, illness, institutionalization (including hospitals!), air pollution, drugs, chemicals, depleted soils, premature harvesting, lengthy transportation of produce, and excess use of water, heat, pressure, and time in food production, to name some of the most important.

Now, national health organizations are sounding a new alarm: Beware of supplement overdose! The truth is that no commonly used drugs can equal the safety and effectiveness of nutritional compounds. All the toxic reactions ever reported for *all* the vitamins used by Americans, for *all* the years these reactions have been documented, amount to less than the toxic reactions reported every year for *each* of the ten drugs most commonly used in America. In fact, in 1985 alone over 3,000 deaths occurred in people taking the

prescribed dose of the right drug for their condition. No unnecessary trage-
dies like these can be attributed to nutritional supplements.

Vitamins can be beneficial in the treatment of virtually all chronic diseases,
even diseases for which no effective drugs are yet known. In fact, vitamins
in sufficient doses, taken under the supervision of care givers trained in
nutrition, can help you cut down or eliminate some drugs you may be taking.
Don't, however, expect your corner physician to know how to use supplements therapeutically. Physicians who know how to use nutrients to treat
disease have not learned this in medical school, but have had to take seminars
and read books and journals on their own.

When you consider that most vitamins were discovered within the lifetime
of Americans living today, it's no wonder that nutritional medicine is a young
and undogmatic science. You are the test tube. You are unique and will need
to monitor your body's feedback carefully so that you and your care giver can
decide on the appropriate supplements and appropriate doses for you. It
may seem more effort than popping a prescribed pill from the pharmacy and
ignoring the body that pill enters, but we promise that by paying attention
to yourself through your nutritional supplement program, you will be re-
warded with an intimate conversation and awareness of your inner needs the
likes of which you may never have experienced before.

Chapter One:

Breasts

In Brief—Breast Conditions

BENIGN CYSTS

Symptoms—Painful mass or masses in one or both breasts.

Signs—Masses easily palpable. Size and tenderness of masses fluctuate, especially during menstrual cycle. Nipple discharge possible.

Cause—Unknown.

Due to—Unknown, though a hormonal influence is suspected. Masses seem to be sensitive to dietary fat, alpha tocopherol (vitamin E). May also be worsened by methylxanthines in coffee, cola, and chocolate.

Solution—Reduce fat in diet, eliminate dairy products, eliminate sugar, increase whole grains and vegetables, reduce or eliminate meat, take supplements, use a brassiere for support both day and night.

Supplements—Vitamin E (mixed tocopherols), selenium, B complex or brewer's yeast, thyroid glandular extract, potassium iodide.

CANCER

Symptoms—Single, firm mass with ill-defined perimeter that does not fluctuate with menstrual cycle, and is usually not painful. May be detected by mammography before a mass can be felt with the fingers. Nipple or skin retraction may be evident.

Signs—Cancer confirmed by laboratory analysis (biopsy) of mass.

Cause—Genetic destruction within breast cells leads to unregulated, disorderly growth uncontrolled by the usual immune defense mechanisms.

Due to—Combination of factors, including environmental chemical toxins, radiation, hormonal stimulation, genetic predisposition, a diet heavy in animal fat and low in antioxidant vitamins and minerals, and long-term emotional trauma.

Solution—Reduce or eliminate environmental toxins (occupation-related, used in home and garden, or in food); reduce dietary fat and increase vitamin- and mineral-rich foods; transform toxic attitudes and emotions to life-enhancing attitudes; surgically remove cancerous tumor.

Supplements—Vitamin A, vitamin E, vitamin C, selenium, multimineral, multivitamin, potassium iodide.

BENIGN CYSTS

Mammary dysplasia, chronic cystic mastitis, and fibrocystic breast disease are terms referring to noncancerous masses in the breast. These benign but distressing masses occur in as many as one in every five American women between the ages of 25 and 50. These masses are sometimes so painful, that the sufferer cannot tolerate anyone touching her breasts, and must wear a bra even to bed to maintain support. In other women, the masses fluctuate in size and tenderness from month to month, becoming most severe the week before menstruation. Commonly, there are multiple masses in both breasts. The condition rarely occurs in women past menopause, suggesting that the problem is related to hormones, particularly estrogen levels.

The risk of breast cancer for women suffering from cystic mastitis is up to eight times that of women free of the condition. If you suffer from breast cysts, please read the section of this chapter on breast cancer prevention.

Some researchers diagnose different breast symptoms as the signs of a wide variety of distinct conditions. Others subsume all breast symptoms under a single term, benign breast disease. The condition is certainly a perplexing one for the orthodox physician. The cause is not known, and there is no cure known to drug-oriented physicians. This frustrating situation has inspired some outrageous sledge-hammer "cures," including surgical removal of the breast. Unfortunately, not even this radical treatment works, since the patient is likely to continue to complain of pain in the area even after surgery.

Another treatment that we consider inappropriate includes the drug Danazol, a synthetic steroid hormone that inhibits release of sex hormones and can cause flushing, sweating, vaginal dryness, reduction in breast size, acne, and facial hair. We also do not recommend megadoses of vitamin A. In one study, 150,000 I.U. of vitamin A were given daily to women suffering from breast cysts, compared to our recommendation of a daily intake of 25,000 I.U. After three months a majority of the patients in the study did enjoy a marked lessening of pain, and 40 percent had measurable reduction of the lumps. But there was no change in the abnormal breast tissue itself. The only toxic effect of this massive dose was a dryness of skin and mucous membranes, which disappeared after vitamin A was discontinued.[1] Nevertheless, we feel that a cure for this condition is possible without super doses of potentially toxic supplements. There are safe and effective treatments, involving a change in diet and modest supplementation of one or more nutrients, that can eliminate both the pain and the cysts.

Vitamin E is the winner as the most useful curative agent. Not only does it eliminate pain and cysts in the majority of women participating in studies using this therapy, it also normalizes hormonal and lipoprotein levels. Because these levels are contributing factors in the development of cancer, vitamin E may be an important aid in cancer prevention.

The amount of the vitamin used in various research and clinical settings has varied from 300 I.U. to 1,200 I.U. daily. Even the lowest doses have led, for some women, to dramatic improvement in a matter of weeks. Dr. Nancy Goldman of West Los Angeles, California, has her patients regulate their own dosage. If a woman takes too little, the lumps and pain persist. If she takes too much she may find her face becoming a bit oily, Goldman says. However, what is too much for one woman may bring soft skin and a gleaming complexion to another, in addition to eliminating her breast cysts. "Vitamin E works!" says Goldman, who uses the vitamin to treat her own cysts.

The first reports of the benefits of vitamin E for breast lumps appeared in 1965, when Dr. Archie A. Abrams of the Boston University School of Medicine, published the results of his research in the *New England Journal of Medicine*. More recently, Dr. Robert S. London and colleagues at the Divisions of Clinical Research and of Clinical Laboratories and Reproductive Endocrinology at Sinai Hospital, Baltimore, have found that up to 85 percent of their patients treated with alpha tocopherol (vitamin E) experienced pain relief and decreased breast lumps.

None of the studies we've read have mentioned timing of the vitamin dose as a relevant factor. Santa Monica naturopath Janet Zand has found that most patients respond more quickly if they take their vitamin E at night. She isn't sure why this is so.

Not *all* women obtain relief simply from swallowing vitamin E. Health problems rarely can be attributed to the lack of a single nutrient and may not be cured by one small change in a generally unhealthy life-style. For example, in the Ohio State University study of the connection between methylxanthines and breast lumps described below, three of seven women whose lumps and pain didn't diminish when they gave up coffee *did* find relief when they also gave up cigarettes.[2]

One Lump or Two? The Coffee Connection

You may have read in the popular press about coffee as a stimulant for mental functions and as a cause of fibrocystic breasts as well. The coffee–breast cyst connection is clear-cut for some women and nonexistent for others. One study of over 850 women with benign breast disease concluded that there was no association between consumption of coffee, tea, cola, and chocolate (all contain caffeine) and the development of cysts. However, In *Medical Makeover*, Dr. Robert M. Giller describes an Ohio State University study conducted by Dr. John Minton in which 65 percent of the women who completely eliminated coffee from their diet were free of breast cysts within six months.[3] Giller has seen similar success among his own patients. So has obstetrician-gynecologist Goldman. Eliminating coffee, she has found, is directly related to reducing the pain of the cysts during the premenstrual week, not only for her patients and her office staff, but for herself as well.

Dr. Minton suggests that a chemical in coffee, called methylxanthine, is to blame for stimulating the development of breast cysts. Why and how still isn't known. There are several kinds of methylxanthines. One methylxanthine found in coffee, some teas, and colas is called caffeine. The methylxanthine in chocolate, some teas, and some soft drinks is theobromine. There is a third methylxanthine, called theophylline and found in tea, which is used by asthmatics to improve their breathing. Minton suggests that methylxanthines stimulate some women's breast cells to develop into cysts, while other cells develop the unregulated and wild growth we call cancer. Unfortunately for coffee lovers, even decaffeinated coffee contains the chemical.

Selenium

Although selenium hasn't been used to eliminate breast cysts as has vitamin E, studies in both Japan and the United States document significantly lower blood selenium levels in women with cystic breasts, levels similar to those found in women with breast cancer. This indicates that adequate selenium definitely plays a part in a breast cancer or breast cyst prevention program.[4]

Relief from the Sea: the Iodine Connection

Dr. Bernard A. Eskin and his colleagues in the departments of obstetrics and gynecology, medicine, and pathology at Women's Medical College of Pennsylvania in Philadelphia gave estrogen to iodine-deficient rats who were lacking thyroid hormone. The rats developed changes in their breasts that resembled human cystic disease. Eskin points out that persons living in areas of normal iodine availability show lower breast cancer rates than those living in areas of low iodine availability. Since cancer occurs more often in breasts with cysts than in normal breasts, he suggests that iodine deficiency, coupled with estrogen stimulation and low thyroid hormone, may all profoundly influence the development of human fibrocystic breast disease and, ultimately, breast cancer. Others, notably Dr. Richard Kunin of San Francisco, a past president of the Orthomolecular Medical Society, uses potassium iodide. We have also found this prescription source of iodine extremely useful. Ask your doctor for SSKI (which stands for supersaturated potassium iodide).

Some gynecologists urge their patients to include iodized salt in their daily meals as an easy way of adding iodine. Another way is to add kelp powder or flakes, purchased in a health-food store, to your food as a substitution for salt. Kelp is a sea plant rich in minerals and iodine.

Seafoods are a good protein source for women with breast cysts, as they also provide iodine and minerals. Cold-water fish like halibut, cod, or salmon also provide the benefit of fish oils, now known to help keep heart disease at bay.

Some researchers have suggested that thyroid hormone can lessen the pain and soften the lumps of fibrocystic breast disease. If you find that you have a chronically low body temperature, it might be an indication that you are hypothyroid. Our recommended procedure for taking your temperature, as well as information on treatment options for hypothyroidism, can be found on page 35.

. . . And the Diet

To be healthy, we need to eliminate unhealthy elements from our lives. Throwing away coffee and cigarettes is a giant improvement. But what we *do* consume is just as important as what we don't. More healthy people around the world eat a diet that is low in fat, sugar, and refined foods, and high in fibers—vegetables, fruits, and whole grains. The more natural the source of your foods, the more these foods can contribute to your health. If you tend to eat out of boxes and cans, consider making a major revision of your diet.

Most meat is polluted with the hormones that are used by ranchers as growth stimulants. The last thing a woman concerned about breast cysts and possibly breast cancer needs is residues of growth hormones lodging in her breast tissue for years. To keep your diet low in animal protein, substitute cold-water fish and high-protein vegetable combinations like corn and beans, or sesame seeds and brown rice. Such a diet will help heal breast disease and improve your overall health.

Brewer's yeast is a food supplement we find especially noteworthy. It is rich in chromium, which helps regulate your appetite, and the all-important B complex vitamins, as well as other important minerals. The B complex, with special mention of vitamin B-6, is especially important for those whose breast pain is part of a general premenstrual syndrome. (See Chapter 5 for a detailed discussion of that monthly scourge.)

At the Douglass Center for Nutrition and Preventive Medicine in Marietta, Georgia, Dr. William C. Douglass gives patients 500 mg of vitamin B-1 (thiamin) twice a day as part of his treatment for breast swelling and pain. Tincture of iodine, thyroid (if indicated), and vitamin E are also part of his breast treatment program. Many women are concerned about yeast infections and may avoid brewer's yeast for fear of encouraging systemic Candida albicans (yeast) growth. We don't believe that taking brewer's yeast will exacerbate Candida growth. But if an individual isn't improving on an anti-Candida diet and is still taking brewer's yeast, she can eliminate the yeast and obtain her vitamin B complex elsewhere, taking a "yeast-free" B complex vitamin each day.

Scientific studies support our conviction that dietary fat is a negative factor, especially for women suffering breast pain. Researchers at the American Health Foundation in New York found that women who adhered to a diet in which a maximum of 20 percent of total calories was fat had markedly reduced breast pain and, in addition, reduced serum estrogen and prolactin levels, serum cholesterol, and body weight. As we discuss in the following section, on cancer, dietary fat reduction is an important part of a cancer prevention program. In fact, a number of studies conclude that high dietary fat encourages the conversion of precancerous growths into malignant tumors in the breast, while depressing the immune response—a particularly dangerous combination.

Our advice is to eat a lot of low-fat, nutrient-rich green and orange vegetables, whole grains such as brown rice and millet, seafoods and seaweeds, and nuts and seeds, and choose 100 percent whole-wheat bakery products for sandwiches and treats. Your breasts—and your whole body—will let you know you've made the right choice.

CANCER

Cancer is a catchall word for malignant tumors. Both benign and malignant tumors are called neoplasms. A growth is considered cancerous if there is an uncontrolled multiplication of cells. DNA, the core genetic material of a cell, becomes damaged by toxins or radiation, and as the cell reproduces, it passes on to its daughter cells incorrect information. Normal cells reproduce throughout life, to repair injured or worn-out tissues and to provide for growth of the body. Once repair or appropriate reproduction occurs, the cell stops dividing. Neoplasms, however, grow uncontrolled until they interfere with normal body processes. If the growth is malignant, the cancer metastasizes, that is, sends malignant cells to other parts of the body, frequently to organs far from the original tumor location, and new tumors start to grow.

There are numerous kinds of cancer, and each has its own appearance and growth pattern. All interfere with the normal functioning of the body by physical obstruction, pressure, or destruction of healthy tissue. Cancer can be initiated by some environmental agents, and is stimulated to keep growing by others. Tumor initiators include ultraviolet radiation, asbestos, DES (diethylstilbestrol), tobacco smoke, pesticides (malathion, DDT), tannic acid, PCBs (polychlorinated biphenyls) and nitrosamines. Tumor promoters include sex steroids, phenobarbital, sodium lauryl sulfate, estrogen, excess fat, and saccharine.[5] Since 80 to 90 percent of all cancers are caused by environmental factors, it can be said that cancer is by and large a preventable disease.

It is also important to understand that throughout our lives we all develop abnormal cells that begin to become cancerous. When our immune system is strong, these abnormal cells are destroyed before they cause too much damage. This means that within each of us is the power to destroy cancerous cells. Women who are treated for breast cancer and whose cancer "goes into remission"—their cancer has disappeared and they lead healthy lives—have restimulated their immune systems to protect themselves from recurrence of the disease. Actually, the idea of "spontaneous remission" is a preposterous insult to the hard work that these patients must do to make that change.

All human beings, except for the few born with missing immune functions, who are destined to live in sterile bubbles, have the capability of healing themselves from cancer. Destroying cancerous cells is an everyday, ordinary, unspectacular function of our immune system. Making the changes necessary to strengthen or regenerate that immune system, however, takes thought, effort, and a fighting spirit.

Thus, if you develop breast cancer and have a mastectomy, a lumpectomy, radiation, or chemotherapy treatment, this treatment is only part of the whole cancer cure. The final half of therapy is to stimulate and regenerate your immune system so that it does the job it was created to do. A part of this regeneration process has to include some careful reflection, not only on the toxic environmental agents that might still be poisoning you—what you eat, drink, wear, inhale, and use each day—but also the thoughts that may be poisoning you.

The Diet-Cancer Connection

Recently, Americans were shocked to learn that the death rate from breast cancer rose 7 percent in one year in women less than 55 years old. As awful as this figure is, there is also good news from medical research: It is now accepted that up to 60 percent of cancers in women are diet-related.

For women, breast cancer is the most frequently diagnosed cancer (26 percent of all cancers). The second most frequent sites are the colon and rectum (15 percent). It seems logical that colon cancer is connected to what you eat—but breast cancer?

Every major health research and health information organization, including the National Research Council, the American Cancer Society, and the American Health Foundation, believes that high consumption of fat contributes to the development of breast cancer.

In the United States today, fat comprises about 40 to 50 percent of our daily caloric intake. These groups suggest that we lower our fat intake to less than 30 percent of our total daily calories; some researchers point to intake rates as low as 10 to 20 percent among populations with very low incidence of breast cancer.[6]

A significant portion of Americans' fat intake is from animals. Avocados, for example, are rich in fat, but we rarely make avocados a central feature of a meal! Animals, including humans, store in fat cells materials the body cannot immediately use, including toxic substances that the body cannot immediately eliminate. A woman who eats fatty meats is consuming, along with the protein, vitamins, and minerals, a portion of the pesticides and herbicides used on the animal's feed, and a portion of the drugs given to the animal during its life to prevent disease or stimulate growth. These toxic substances are then concentrated in the woman's own fat cells. Breasts are to a large extent "adipose tissue," or fat. So a woman's breasts are storehouses of numerous toxic substances from up and down the food chain.

Some studies indicate that women who are obese have a higher incidence of breast cancer than those who are not overweight. Obesity may be a risk factor for breast cancer, not only because of the increased volume of toxins, but also because fat tissue can convert androgens to estrogens (we explain this process in detail in Chapter 11, on menopause). This increase in circulating estrogens may affect the body's endocrine system and stimulate the development of a tumor. It is known, for example, that women who begin menstruating before age 12 and/or go through menopause after age 50 have a higher risk of breast cancer, suggesting that lengthened years of hormonal stimulation also has something to do with cancer risk.

In addition to concentrating toxic substances, dietary fat stimulates secretion of the hormone prolactin by the pituitary gland. This hormone is known to promote breast cancer in rats, although its relationship to human breast cancer has not been confirmed.

There probably are other reasons why high-fat diets lead to an increased incidence of breast cancer, but these reasons are unknown at this time. The fat–cancer relationship is very strong, however. The graph on page 25 shows the correlation between per capita consumption of dietary fat in 40 countries and age-related deaths from breast cancer. Within the United States, Seventh Day Adventists have lower cancer rates than usual in the general population. Members of this religious group consume significantly less meat and more foods rich in vitamins A and C than the general American population. Japanese women in Japan have a very low incidence of breast and colon cancer, while stomach cancer there is a more frequent occurrence, which has been attributed to the importance of pickled foods in the Japanese diet. When those women come to the United States, the pattern shifts, which can be seen most clearly after two or three generations grow up in America: The incidence of stomach cancer drops and that of breast and colon cancer rises. Why? As Japanese women change their diet to the Standard American Diet (SAD), their intake of pickled foods decreases and their intake of foods laden with animal fat and additives increases. Researchers at the University of California at Berkeley found a similar development in Chinese-American women. Chinese-American women with breast cancer ate a more Westernized diet, consuming less fish and chicken and more beef and pork than cancer-free Chinese-American women.

Other probable dietary factors contributing to the development of breast cancer are excess protein intake, which goes along with excess animal fat intake, and insufficient dietary fiber, which also goes along with overindulgence in meat and consumption of too few vegetables and whole grains.

Vitamins and minerals play an important but complicated role in cancer prevention. Their usefulness centers around their ability to protect the body from the ravages of substances called "free radicals." A free radical usually is a fragment of an oxygen molecule that has an unpaired "free" electron. This makes the fragment highly unstable and extremely eager to link up with anything it can latch on to. What it usually finds to attach itself to are cell membranes or fat molecules. Rancidity is the result of the deterioration free radicals cause in oils and fats. Unfortunately, when a free radical attaches itself to the fat within your cell membranes, your body is the material that deteriorates.

Free radicals are produced by ordinary metabolic processes, or are consumed in foods, such as the black part of charcoal-broiled meat. Our body protects us from these harmful free radicals by producing enzymes such as

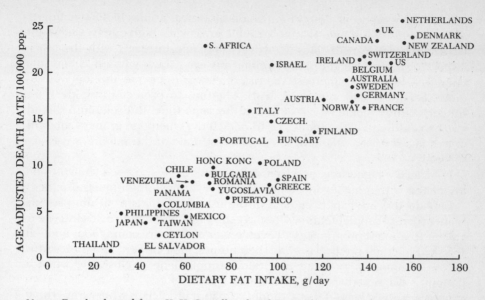

AGE-ADJUSTED DEATH RATE/100,000 pop. vs DIETARY FAT INTAKE, g/day

NETHERLANDS
UK
CANADA • DENMARK
S. AFRICA • NEW ZEALAND
SWITZERLAND
IRELAND • US
ISRAEL
BELGIUM
AUSTRALIA
SWEDEN
AUSTRIA • GERMANY
NORWAY • FRANCE
ITALY
CZECH.
FINLAND
PORTUGAL HUNGARY
HONG KONG • POLAND
CHILE
BULGARIA
VENEZUELA → ROMANIA SPAIN
GREECE
PANAMA YUGOSLAVIA
PUERTO RICO
COLUMBIA
PHILIPPINES MEXICO
JAPAN • TAIWAN
CEYLON
THAILAND EL SALVADOR

NOTE: Graph adapted from K. K. Carroll and and H. T. Khor, "Dietary Fat in Relation to Tumorigenesis," *Progressive Biochemical Pharmacology* 10 (1975), 308. Reproduced by permission of S. Karger AG, Basel.

superoxide dismutase and glutathione peroxidase, that destroy free radicals. Certain vitamins and minerals found in foods do a good job of scavenging the wild molecules, too. These vitamins and minerals are called antioxidants, since they oppose the process of oxidation caused by the wayward oxygen fragments. These antioxidants are the vitamins A, C, and E, and the mineral selenium.

Certain vitamins also prevent the formation of cancer-causing substances in your body. If you eat nitrite- or nitrate-containing foods such as bacon, sausage, hot dogs, or bologna, be sure to eat vitamin C– and E–containing foods or take supplements of these vitamins at the same meal. In your stomach, nitrates turn into nitrites, and nitrites in the presence of food substances called amines turn into nitrosamines, which are potentially cancer-causing toxins. Vitamins C and E protect your stomach, colon, and bladder from the nitrosamines.[7]

These vitamins also help reduce levels of other mutagenic substances (those causing genetic changes in cells that may lead to cancer), both cancer initiators and cancer promoters. Vitamins C, E, A, and D have the power to convert cancer cells back to healthy cells and to stimulate the immune system to destroy those cancer cells not converted. Beta carotene, a precursor for vitamin A, has its own cancer-inhibiting and cancer-preventing powers.[8]

Deficiencies of vitamin A, vitamin C, vitamin E, and selenium are all associated with a higher incidence of cancer. The breast cancer–selenium connection is especially important; epidemiological studies in different parts of the world have shown that geographic areas with high dietary selenium have low breast cancer rates. However, selenium interacts with the other important anticancer nutrients in different ways: Low vitamin E and low vitamin A levels both increase the risk of cancer in people also low in selenium. Selenium and vitamin A work together to protect the body from cancer, so they should be consumed at the same time. But selenium should *not* be consumed with vitamin C: In one study, when one gram of vitamin C was taken with a selenium source, almost none of the selenium was absorbed.

Folic acid, magnesium, and iron deficiencies have also been shown to be associated with a higher incidence of cancer, as have high levels of zinc.

Few doctors are expert enough in the use of nutrients as healing agents to incorporate supplements of vitamins, minerals, and amino acids into their cancer treatment programs. And even fewer doctors are courageous enough to risk losing their medical license, their homes, their careers, and their status in the community by using nutritional supplements exclusively, when a patient is diagnosed as having cancer.

In fact, it could be said that a vendetta against physicians who use anything other than radiation, chemotherapy, or surgery is now in progress. A number of physicians have already lost their licenses to practice medicine in their home states, not because any patient complained, but because it became known to the state medical board that their treatment included "unorthodox" methods of helping the body heal itself. Of course, radiation, chemotherapy, and surgery do nothing to help the body heal itself. The best these treatments can do is remove enough of an invasive tumor to buy time for the body's own healing powers to do *their* work. But the powerful state boards of medical quality assurance, along with the state medical associations and the American Medical Association (A.M.A), have limited the acceptable medical treatment for cancer to those three techniques and are vigorously prosecuting anyone who dares to use his or her own methods, whether or not those methods work.

Consequently, in this book we are not going to describe a nutrient-based cancer treatment program. The organizations listed under For Further Information will refer you to metabolic nutrition–oriented physicians in your area. We *are* going to describe a cancer *prevention* program; such a program is equally important for those who have already been treated for breast cancer and for those who have had no experience with breast cancer.

We do want to mention that vitamins A, C, and E have played an important role in many cancer therapies supervised by nutrition-aware physicians. Vitamin C, for example, has been used by Dr. Ewan Cameron, a Scottish physician and researcher who is currently the medical director and senior research professor at the Linus Pauling Institute of Science and Medicine in Palo Alto, California. Although Dr. Cameron states categorically that vitamin C is not of itself a cure for cancer, he has for many years witnessed a restoration of energy, activity, and a general sense of well being, as well as increased survival rates, in patients given supplemental ascorbic acid. Cameron explains that the vitamin C supplements become involved in a biochemical reaction that transforms the amino acid lysine to an amino-acid-like substance called carnitine.

Carnitine has been called "a nutritional moving van" and "the biochemical carburetor" because it carries fatty acids and triglycerides, our body's "fuel," through the mitochondrial membrane into the mitochondria within a cell, our "engine," where the fatty acids and triglycerides are burned for energy. The body cannot use fat for energy without adequate carnitine, and the amount of carnitine available is limited by the amount of vitamin C available. Since breast cancer risk is connected to fat, it is in your best interest to metabolize fat as efficiently as possible. Thus, carnitine and vitamin C play an important role in cancer prevention. And in cases of active cancer, vitamin C supplementation, by increasing the amount of carnitine in the body, helps prevent the atrophying of muscles from disuse, weight loss, and the lethargy that often accompany long-term cancer illness.[9]

One further supplement we recommend is coenzyme Q, an excellent immune system stimulant that takes part in a multitude of metabolic reactions. Coenzyme Q has proven useful in the treatment of a wide range of conditions, including cancer. It is in the same family of substances as vitamin K. Also, just as with cysts, potassium iodide is useful for breast cancer prevention and nutritional support.

How Supplements Help

Patients who are undergoing traditional, orthodox treatment for breast cancer will be delighted to know that supplementation of vitamin A and vitamin E enhances the beneficial effects of radiation and chemotherapy and minimizes side effects such as hair loss and heart disease. Sixteen hundred I.U. of vitamin E (d-alpha tocopherol acetate) was given to patients a week before these patients received doxorubicin (Adriamycin), a chemotherapeutic drug. Sixty-nine percent of these patients did not lose their hair, and those who did were believed to have been given the vitamin E too late before chemotherapy started.

The results of research with vitamin C (ascorbic acid, or ascorbate) and cancer treatment are mixed, depending on the type of tumor and the drug used. Folic acid, a B-complex vitamin, was found to increase the toxicity of 5-fluorouracil, a chemotherapeutic agent, and caused severe enough reactions that the researchers warned against future use of the supplement in studies on humans.

Prevention Is Part of Every Treatment

Women who have had cancer in one breast are at high risk of developing it in the other one. We look at cancer as a multicausal disease, created by environmental toxins that possibly combine with toxic emotional attitudes. Over the years, toxins eat away at a woman until her body's physical defenses are overwhelmed. Thus, it makes perfect sense that a cancer that is simply removed, without paying attention to the causes, will recur. A woman who begins a self-care program like the one outlined below will be doing everything she possibly can to live a long, cancer-free life, whether she has ever developed cancer in the past or not.

In almost every case of cancer, a woman goes to a physician for an evaluation of a lump that she or her partner has found in her breast. The lump is usually not painful. It is a firm mass with vague borders, and is almost half the time found in the outer quadrant of the breast (the area from the nipple up to the underarm). Occasionally, there will be nipple discharge or some change in the nipple, or a physical change in color or texture of the breast. Only about 15 percent of breast cancers occur in premenopausal women. Since cancer does, however, sometimes occur in women well under 50, most medical authorities recommend all women to check their own breasts each month.

The best time to check for breast lumps is a few days after menstrual bleeding ends, as this is the time when any cysts that come and go with the menstrual period will be minimal. Postmenopausal women can choose a set day, such as the first of the month. If you need education about breast self-examination, the American Cancer Society offers printed material and training. You may want to add breast self-examination to your cancer-prevention program.

Our basic cancer-prevention self-care program emphasizes the following:

· Eat nutritious food. A healthy diet is low in fat and includes frequent servings of cruciferous vegetables (cauliflower, broccoli, brussels sprouts) and vitamin A–rich and carotene-rich foods (sweet potatoes, carrots, winter squash, cantaloupe, dark-green leafy vegetables, tomatoes and strawberries). Surprisingly, a correlation has been found between consumption of tomatoes and strawberries and low cancer risk, while no correlation has been found between consumption of salads, carrots, and squash and cancer risk. Yet overall, people who ate the greatest quantity of carotene-rich vegetables, that is, the green and orange ones, had only one third the cancer mortality of those who ate the smallest quantities of these foods.[10] The fiber present in whole grains and a vegetarian diet also seems to encourage the removal of estrogen through the feces, reducing the risk of hormonal stimulation of tumors.

  Rather than go all-out vegetarian, you may want to eat several fish meals per week, or take supplemental omega-3 fatty acids, available in health-food stores as Max-EPA. Animal studies indicate that this fish oil may inhibit the development of breast cancer.

· Eliminate sugar from your diet. Animal and human research indicates a definite correlation between sugar consumption and breast cancer. One study that included data from 21 countries reveals that sugar intake is a major risk factor in the development of breast cancer in women older than 45.[11]

· Avoid eating any food that has hydrogenated or partially hydrogenated oil listed as an ingredient. Even health-food store sweets frequently list partially hydrogenated oils on their label. The unnatural "trans" form of the fatty acid in these oils is suspected of causing cancer.[12]

· Drink unpolluted water. Install a reverse osmosis filtration system in your home if you can afford it, or use less expensive, and less effective, alternatives if you can't, such as carbon block filters, or at the very least, bottled water, either home-delivered from a bottler or purchased at the supermarket. Tap water is one of the most common sources of toxic industrial and agricultural chemicals and heavy metals (such as lead) that poison Americans.[13]

· Take regular aerobic exercise. Walking is good enough, if you don't care to bicycle, jog, run, swim, skate, or dance. This improves blood and lymph circulation, helps maintain proper weight, and stimulates the release of endorphins, naturally occurring morphinelike biochemicals that reduce pain and make you feel happy.

· Take time to relax. Relaxation reduces stress, allows body processes to rest and regenerate, and helps you remain resilient in the face of the pressures of life.

· Take supplements of vitamins A, C, and E, magnesium, selenium, and essential fatty acids.[14] The National Academy of Sciences has recommended that people eat vitamin A–rich foods daily to help prevent disease. You can add a natural precursor of vitamin A, called beta carotene, to your diet without fear of the toxic effects of excess vitamin A. The active form of vitamin E is called alpha tocopherol, and is not toxic even in high doses. Vitamin C in high doses can cause abdominal discomfort and diarrhea. This symptom indicates the appropriate individualized dose of the vitamin. Dr. Robert Cathcart of Los Altos, California, is one of the most experienced physicians in using vitamin C therapeutically. He claims when the quantity of the vitamin is so great that it can no longer be absorbed through the lining of the intestine, diarrhea occurs. The sicker the patient, the more vitamin C can be absorbed before this tolerance point is reached. The correct dose of C, then, is discovered by taking just enough to cause diarrhea, then cutting back until no diarrhea occurs.

The minerals magnesium and selenium have been shown to be deficient in the soil and food in areas where cancer mortality is high. Research suggests that 250 to 300 micrograms (mcg) of selenium daily can prevent most cancers. Unfortunately, the average amount of selenium Americans receive in their food is less than 100 mcg daily. Studies of large populations confirm that cancer patients tend to have lower selenium levels in their blood than healthy people. In one study, the serum selenium levels of 35 breast cancer patients were significantly lower than those of healthy controls.

Take vitamins A and E twice a day, morning and evening. Take selenium once a day with vitamin E. Take vitamin C four times a day, since it is so much more quickly eliminated from the body in your urine. Take magnesium once a day, on an empty stomach.

We also advocate using a multimineral and a multivitamin in addition to these individual supplements, to assure yourself of the nutrients your body needs for optimum functioning and healing.

· Provide for adequate iodine. Use iodized salt and kelp powder, include seaweeds in soups, and increase the amount of seafood you eat.

· Check for heavy metal toxicity, especially cadmium, mercury, or aluminum. Dr. James Privitera of Covina, California, has found cadmium toxicity in breast cancer patients and uses such supplements as sulphated amino acids and zinc to draw out the cadmium, among other treatments.

· Give yourself a hefty dose of laughter and optimism every day. Vitamins cannot compensate for a negative attitude! It is of utmost importance for your health to seek out the positives, and include them in your daily life, even as you acknowledge and work to change the political and social evils of our day. Listen to comedy records. Read the funnies in the newspaper. Buy humor books and memorize several jokes a week to brighten the day of those you meet. Share your smile frequently. This isn't frivolous, it is health-enhancing behavior, proven to affect your physiology. Dr. William Fry, an associate clinical professor in the Department of Psychiatry at Stanford University, who has dubbed his specialty gelotology, from the Greek *gelos,* "laughter," and Norman Cousins, former editor of *Saturday Review* and currently adjunct professor at the UCLA School of Medicine, both call laughter "a form of internal jogging."

Daily Supplement Dose Advisory—Breast Conditions

CYSTS

Vitamin E—800 I.U.
B complex—50 to 100 mg of the major B vitamins
Thyroid—take as prescribed by physician
(or Thyroid glandular)—take as directed on label
(or potassium iodide) (SSKI)—½ dropperful 3 times a day in glass of water
Selenium—200 mcg
Carnitine—dose depends on the brand used

CANCER

A—10,000 I.U.
C—to bowel tolerance, beginning with 5000 mg per day in divided doses
E—800 I.U.
selenium—200 mcg
potassium iodide—½ dropperful 3 times a day in glass of water. (If liquid unavailable, use another iodide salt at 150 to 1,000 mg per day depending on individual need. Best to seek professional advice.
magnesium—800 mg
Coenzyme Q—60 mg
multivitamin—A national brand purchased in a health food store, not a drugstore house brand.
multimineral—A product containing trace minerals such as manganese, vanadium, molybdenum.

Chapter Two:
Uterus and Ovaries

In Brief—Uterus and Ovaries

CERVIX

Cervical Dysplasia
Symptoms—None.
Signs—None. Diagnosis is based on laboratory analysis of Pap smear.
Cause—Unknown, but associated with same factors as cervical cancer: earlier age at first intercourse, multiple sexual partners, viral diseases such as genital herpes and genital warts.
Due to—Defect of immune response to repeated exposure to irritating substance which leads to abnormal changes in cells of cervix.
Solution—Change in diet to eliminate sugar, coffee, and refined foods and add whole grains, green and orange vegetables, seeds, and supplements. If severe, removal by cryosurgery, electrocauterization, or laser.
Supplements—Folic acid, B complex or brewer's yeast, vitamin A, vitamin E, vitamin C, a multimineral that includes selenium, magnesium, zinc.

Cervical Cancer
Symptoms—Abnormal uterine bleeding and vaginal discharge.
Signs—Visible tumor or ulceration of cervix and/or laboratory confirmation via biopsy.
Cause—Unknown, but associated with earlier age of intercourse, a higher number of sexual partners, viral diseases such as genital herpes and genital warts, unfulfilled need for love coupled with hopelessness.
Due To—Defective immune response to abnormally replicating cells.
Solution—Change diet as with cervical dysplasia, take supplements, surgery.
Supplements—Folic acid, Vitamin A, Vitamin E, Vitamin C, selenium, multivitamin, multimineral.

UTERUS

Uterine Cancer

Symptoms—Excessive bleeding before, during, or after menstruation or spotting postmenopausally; lower abdominal cramps.

Signs—Dilation and curettage (D&C) allows laboratory analysis of tissues for diagnosis.

Cause—Unknown, but clearly an increase in estrogens is involved, coupled with overload of toxicity and inability of body to remove waste adequately.

Due to—Postmenopausal estrogen replacement therapy, obesity, hypertension, diabetes, polycystic ovarian syndrome.

Solution—Halt use of supplemental estrogens; maintain proper body weight; lower blood pressure; heal ovaries; change diet, including more iodine-rich foods; take supplements; handle life-style stresses.

Supplements—Vitamin A, vitamin C, vitamin E, selenium, multivitamin, multimineral.

OVARIES

Ovarian Cysts

Symptoms—There may be no symptoms, or there may be aching pelvic pain, painful intercourse, and pain when the ovary is touched during a pelvic exam.

Signs—Small cysts may be felt during pelvic examination. Larger cysts may cause bloating of the abdomen, and be diagnosed from other conditions only by ultrasonogram or surgery (laparotomy, laparoscopy, or culdoscopy). With polycystic ovarian disease (Stein-Leventhal Syndrome), there may also be infertility and amenorrhea, or lack of menstruation.

Cause—Unknown. We believe a toxic body and hormonal imbalances contribute to the condition.

Due to—Environmental pollutants, improper diet, nutritional deficiencies, emotional stress.

Solution—Rebalance body chemistry through change in diet, nutritional supplements, stress reduction, and detoxification.

Supplements—Vitamin E, vitamin B complex, thyroid.

Ovarian Cancer

Symptoms—Commonly there are no symptoms; there may be nonspecific pelvic discomfort or swelling in advanced cases.

Signs—Enlargement found during routine pelvic examination, enlarged abdomen or difficulty breathing due to fluid accumulation.

Cause—Not known.

Due to—Since the disease is associated with a high-fat diet, beginning menstruation at a young age, few or no children, and later age at marriage, there seems to be a connection with years of exposure to estrogen, coupled with depressed immune system.

Solution—Prevention involves changing diet, taking supplements, resolving relationship problems, and eliminating toxic substances and thoughts. Treatment involves same steps as prevention, in addition to whatever treatment your oncologist and you decide upon.
Supplements—Vitamin A, vitamin C, vitamin E, selenium, multivitamin, multimineral.

CERVIX

Cervical Dysplasia

Dysplasia means disordered growth. The term cervical dysplasia refers to abnormal cell growth on areas of the cervix, the neck of the uterus, which juts into the vagina. These areas may be mildly, moderately, or severely abnormal. It is generally believed that dysplasia can progress to an even more severe disorganization of the cells in a particular area, called carcinoma in situ, which may, if conditions do not change, progress to invasive cancer in about a third of these cases. Severe dysplasia progresses to cancer more frequently and more rapidly than mild dysplasia. Oral contraceptives are suspected of accelerating this unhealthy development.

The cause of dysplasia is unknown. Certain social factors seem to be associated with the condition, the same as are associated with cervical cancer. Sexual activity is strongly connected to the appearance of unhealthy changes in the cervix. Both dysplasia and cancer are unusual in celibate women or lesbians, but are more common in women who had their first intercourse as a teenager. Jewish women of any sexual history have a much lower incidence than other groups. Whether this is due to hereditary immunity or better hygiene isn't clear. Dysplasia is also associated with viral diseases such as genital herpes or genital warts. Women with genital herpes, for example, are six times more likely to develop dysplasia than women who do not have herpes.

Women whose mothers took the drug diethylstilbestrol (DES) when pregnant with them are at great risk of developing cervical dysplasia and are among those recommended to have regular Pap (Papanicolaou) smear examinations to catch any abnormalities early.

One to 4 percent of nonpregnant gynecology patients test positive for cervical dysplasia, the greatest number of cases occurring between ages 25 and 35.

Eliminating Dysplasia Through Supplements

Treatment is too frequently limited to simply removing the offending abnormal tissues with cryosurgery (freezing), electrocauterization (burning), or laser surgery (cutting) without changing any of the conditions that contributed to their development. Thus it isn't surprising that at least 10 percent of cases recur after such treatments. What is surprising is how many medical textbooks say nothing about eliminating toxins, supplementing the diet with cancer-healing and cancer-preventing nutrients, and changing the diet from a carcinogenic one to a health-promoting one.

Folic acid supplementation has been shown to eliminate even moderately severe dysplasia and to reduce the progression to carcinoma in situ. In a five-year study by Dr. C. E. Butterworth of the University of Alabama School of Medicine in Birmingham and the Contraceptive Evaluation Branch, National Institute of Child Health and Human Development, Bethesda, Maryland, 10 mg of folate daily for three months was enough to significantly improve or eliminate the condition, while none of the controls receiving a placebo improved. Seven of the women receiving folate were completely cured of their dysplasia. None receiving folate progressed to carcinoma in situ, while four women receiving a placebo did progress to the more serious condition. Researchers found lower blood concentrations of folic acid among oral contraceptive users than nonusers, and the lowest measures were among those oral contraceptive users who exhibited cervical dysplasia.[1] In another study, changes of cervical cells in women using oral contraceptives disappeared after the women took folic acid supplements, even though the researchers could find no evidence that these women's folic acid levels were significantly lower than normal.

Even before Butterworth and his team made their important discoveries of the usefulness of folic acid, another group of researchers had documented lower vitamin C intake among women with cervical dysplasia than in controls. Using a three-day food analysis, the vitamin C content of foods eaten by 29 percent of the women suffering cervical dysplasia was less than half of the Recommended Dietary Allowance, compared to only 3 percent of the controls.

Follow-up studies confirmed this vitamin C–dysplasia connection.[2] Indeed, vitamin C is a standard addition to any healing regimen. It ups your immune function and lowers your risk for cancer and viral conditions. Vitamin C is required for many, many chemical reactions in the body. Vitamin C not only increases the number of lymphocytes, the specialized defense cells that fight invaders, but also increases the quantity of a certain protein substance in blood called "complement," which combines with antibodies to eliminate malignancies. The vitamin also increases levels of interferon, our body's homemade virus fighter.

The folic acid researchers wondered about the relationship between folic acid and vitamin C. They analyzed the folic acid *and* vitamin C content of commonly eaten foods, and found that there is a highly significant correlation. In other words, women low in one of these nutrients are likely to be low in the other. Thus, Butterworth and colleagues suggest that "both folic acid and vitamin C are involved in the pathogenesis of cervical dysplasia by mechanisms that are not well understood at this time."

Vitamin A is especially important to the health of the mucous membranes. In one research study, vitamin A and beta-carotene levels in 49 women with cervical dysplasia or carcinoma in situ were measured and compared to 49 controls. The results suggested that women who consume below-average quantities of vitamin A and beta-carotene were 3 times as likely to develop severe dysplasia and 2¾ times as likely to develop carcinoma in situ. Other research has confirmed the connection between vitamin A and its precursor, beta carotene, and cervical dysplasia.[3]

Since vitamin E helps the body use vitamin A efficiently, we recommend taking these two nutrients together in cases of cervical dysplasia.

Are You Hypothyroid?

We also suggest that women test their thyroid function, since low thyroid (hypothyroidism) requires extra effort on the part of the pituitary gland to stimulate the thyroid to produce more hormones. But the pituitary also secretes messengers that stimulate the ovaries to produce more estrogen. So hypothyroid women tend to have problems associated with excess estrogen. We feel that any abnormality of the female genital tract may indicate an imbalance of sex hormones and a need for careful rebalancing of these hormones. In addition, the conversion of dietary beta carotene to vitamin A is impaired in cases of hypothyroidism, and since vitamin A helps the body to avoid developing cancer and to heal from cancer, it is quite important to maintain proper thyroid hormone levels.

You can test your own thyroid function. When you go to bed, place a thermometer where it is in easy reach. In the morning, before you say or do anything, place the thermometer in your armpit and wait five to ten minutes. If your temperature is below 97.8° Fahrenheit, you are possibly hypothyroid. Before you rush to your doctor for a prescription for thyroid hormone, take a trip to the health-food store and ask the clerk for a thyroid glandular, which is a product created from animal thyroid-gland material. If, after a couple of weeks of taking the glandular, your temperature doesn't increase above 97.8 degrees and other symptoms don't show signs of improvement, it's time to see your physician to discuss obtaining a prescription for Armour Thyroid or Cytomel, both sources of natural thyroid hormone. We do not recommend Synthroid, the most popular brand prescribed, because it is synthetic and is not as biologically suitable as the natural products.

This simple technique for assessing thyroid function is controversial, and many conventional doctors are unfamiliar with its use and great value. Most doctors are trained to rely only on expensive blood tests of thyroid function, which miss *many* cases of underactive thyroid glands. If your regular doctor should refuse to give you thyroid hormone on the basis of your low underarm temperatures, give your physician a copy of *Hypothyroidism: The Hidden Illness* (see Selected Bibliography) by Dr. Broda O. Barnes and ask her or him to read it. Dr. Barnes makes a very convincing case for the great value of thyroid supplements and underarm temperature testing. Some doctors welcome patients' efforts to expand their awareness of medicine. Do insist on taking Armour thyroid or Cytomel brand, from natural sources, not Synthroid, the synthetic thyroid. If your physician isn't receptive to these ideas, think about finding a more progressive, open-minded physician. In any event, take supplements that combine all of the ingredients needed by your thyroid gland to function well, such as tyrosine, iodine, B-6, and a thyroid glandular. Some patients have had dramatic improvements in their lives just by taking these supplements. Or ask your doctor for a prescription of SSKI (supersaturated potassium iodide), manufactured by Upsher-Smith of Minneapolis. This product may be sufficient without thyroid supplementation.

B vitamins are especially needed in cases of excess estrogen. For example, vitamin B-6 is instrumental in the production of progesterone, the sex hormone that interacts with estrogen: When progesterone levels rise, estrogen levels fall. So, in addition to folic acid supplementation, we recommend taking a good, strong B complex, or supplementing with brewer's yeast, which is rich in B vitamins and useful minerals.

There is a place for mineral supplementation in cases of hypothyroidism and/or abnormal cervical cells. The three most important minerals in cases of cervical dysplasia are selenium, magnesium, and zinc. However, we feel that a multimineral that includes these three nutrients will do an adequate job of raising body stores, rather than your taking three separate minerals each day.

Selenium has been shown to be a critical factor in cancer prevention (see the section on breast cancer in Chapter 1 for more details). To prevent cervical dysplasia from turning into cancer, we recommend selenium supplementation.

Magnesium plays a role in cellular metabolic processes, but also facilitates the body's use of many of the B vitamins, including folic acid. And it activates vitamins C and E. Magnesium is an important coenzyme in the manufacture of sex hormones, and it helps the body eliminate the wastes of protein metabolism. At the cellular level, magnesium converts dietary fat into fatty acids, which are used by cells to build and maintain their membranes.

Zinc is the body's healer. Inadequate zinc leads to poor wound healing and inadequate immune system response to infection. In addition to obtaining zinc from a multimineral, you can raise your zinc stores by eating seaweeds, seafood (especially oysters), eggs, mushrooms, and pumpkin seeds. Vitamin A helps the body absorb zinc, so taking this vitamin with your mineral supplement is a good idea.

Along with supplementation, a change in diet is recommended. Notice what you are eating, drinking, and inhaling that are toxic. Do you use filtered water? Do you choose organic produce if it is available in health-food stores or local farmer's markets? Have you quit smoking cigarettes and drinking coffee? Are you using a protective screen on your video display terminal to eliminate or at least reduce your exposure to the nonionizing radiation emitted from its cathode ray tube?

We recommend you eliminate sugar and white-flour products from your diet completely. Replace the old standbys with whole-grain products from your health-food store. Eat dried fruits or fresh fruits instead of candy. Let raisins soak in water in the refrigerator overnight, and use the liquid instead of sugar for everything from breakfast cereal to baked goods. Spend your money on succulent and exotic varieties of natural foods you ordinarily wouldn't purchase, using the money you have saved by eliminating unnutritious pleasure foods from your weekly menus.

Reduce your intake of fats, especially animal fats. We don't believe that women and dairy products are a good match. Many Asian, black, and Jewish women and some Caucasian women are allergic to cow's milk. Dairy products are high in fat and contribute to congestion of the body with mucus. Many women find that a variety of ailments of the skin, bowel, and respiratory system disappear when they eliminate dairy foods from their diet. As you streamline your own diet to increase the amount of healthy foods and eliminate those that stress your body, we recommend that you slowly replace dairy foods with alternatives such as soy or rice-based ice creams (not Tofutti, however, as this product has precious little soy in it), whipped tofu for sauces, soy milk or almonds blended with water for almond milk. Look in any of dozens of excellent natural foods cookbooks for advice and inspiration.

Cervical Cancer

Statistics on cervical cancer are changing for the worse, with younger women—even teenagers—developing the disease in recent years, although the average age of diagnosis is 45. Where unhealthy changes in the cells of the cervix, as revealed by a Pap smear, previously took five to ten years to develop into cancer, gynecologists are now finding a quicker transformation occurs. They blame these changes on the epidemic of genital warts (human papillomavirus or HPV) that has swept across the country, though there is as yet no definite proof of a cause-effect relationship.

Approximately 16,000 cases of cervical cancer are diagnosed each year in the United States, accounting for about 3 percent of women's deaths from cancer. About a fourth of these cases are in women over age 65. Over 95 percent of cervical cancer is curable if found in its early stages.

Bleeding between menstrual periods and odorous vaginal discharge are common symptoms of cervical cancer. There may also be bleeding after intercourse.

Although the cause of cervical cancer is unknown, certain factors are associated with the disease: virus infections, including the herpes virus as well as venereal warts, and sexual activity. Back in 1842, two Italian doctors first reported a lower cervical cancer rate among nuns, compared to married women. In fact, it is now well accepted that cervical cancer is unknown in celibate women and lesbians, while prostitutes are at four times normal risk for the disease. Jewish women of any sexual history have a lower incidence than other groups. No one knows why, though in the past the reason was thought to be that Jewish men are circumcised. This correlation has repeatedly been proved to be nonexistent.

Some authorities suggest that measures for prevention of cervical cancer includes washing the penis before intercourse and use of a condom, as well as prompt treatment for vaginal and cervical infections of any sort. Removal of venereal warts is also highly recommended, as they are exceedingly contagious, yet easy for a dermatologist or gynecologist to remove by means of a simple office procedure. An annual Pap smear is also recommended, so cervical dysplasia can be diagnosed and treated promptly, before it develops into cancer. These measures are useful, but not enough to prevent dangerous changes in the woman's body if her diet, nutrient intake, and overall lifestyle are health-destroying.

We discuss diet and supplementation for cancer in the section on breast cancer in Chapter 1 and have reiterated some of this information in our discussion of cervical dysplasia. In brief, cancer is a systemic condition, regardless of the site where it is discovered, and it is a sign that the body's internal defense system isn't functioning adequately. It is a warning that a toxic environment, including what the woman eats, drinks, inhales, and feels in personal interactions, is eating away at her from the inside out.

We suggest that any cancer is the outward manifestation of something or several things in the woman's environment or thoughts that are standing in the way of perfect health. Radical methods of eliminating abnormal cells are only a fraction of the whole treatment plan.

Preventing Cervical Cancer

Eliminating health-destroying behavior includes switching from oral contraceptives to a barrier method of birth control, since some studies indicate Pill users develop cervical cancer at a faster rate than nonusers. The condom, and to a lesser extent the cervical cap, protect the cervix from exposure to warts, herpes, trichomonas, and sperm. This is no small detail; a study published nine years ago by researchers at the Kaiser-Permanente Medical Center in Walnut Creek, California, found that cervical cancer is four times lower in women whose sexual partners have had vasectomies (the operation that eliminates sperm from the man's ejaculate).

In our opinion, preventing any kind of cancer most definitely also involves stopping smoking, reducing or eliminating exposure to toxic chemicals and both ionizing and nonionizing radiation, and transforming your diet from one high in sugar, hydrogenated or partially hydrogenated oils and fat to one high in green and orange vegetables (rich in vitamins and minerals), whole grains, seeds, and seafoods (rich in zinc, iodine, and other minerals). We aren't alone in emphasizing the role of nutrition in cancer prevention. Dr. Gio Gori, director of the National Cancer Institute's Diet, Nutrition, and Cancer Program, admitted to Congress over 10 years ago that 50 percent of all human cancers are diet-related, and back in February 1984, the American Cancer Society published specific dietary recommendations for cancer prevention.

Vitamins A, E, and C and selenium are also crucial components of our pro-health, cancer-prevention program. These are the free-radical scavengers of the nutrient family. Free radicals are atoms with unpaired electrons, making them highly reactive. They latch on to unsaturated fats in cell membranes and create, by that new bond, another free radical, which creates yet another in a destructive chain reaction that ends with damage to cells, impairment of function, and carcinogenesis. In our section on breast cancer we describe the usefulness of these nutrients not only to prevent cancer, but to maximize the effectiveness and reduce the toxic side effects of radiation and chemotherapy treatments once the disease exists.

A study of women with cervical cancer, specifically, indicated that women with the lowest percentage of beta carotene in their blood (beta carotene is a vitamin A precursor found in the white of citrus rind, green and leafy vegetables, cantaloupe, strawberries, and orange-fleshed squashes) were four times more likely to have cervical cancer than women with the highest percentage. Overall, women with a high intake of beta carotene–rich food were twice as likely to be cancer-free as those with a low intake. A 1984 study of 191 patients and 191 age-matched controls found that those women who ate a great deal of beta carotene–rich foods were the least likely to develop cervical cancer, while consumption of vitamin A alone as it occurs in milk and meat had no effect on cancer risk. Another study concluded that low blood serum levels of vitamin A may be associated with the development of cervical cancer. We see this as further evidence that a vegetable-based diet is the most healthful a woman can consume.

As for vitamin C, in one experiment plasma vitamin C levels were found to be significantly lower in 78 women with untreated cervical cancer than in the healthy controls. So vitamin C and vitamin A are good choices in a cancer-prevention program.

Returning the body to a state of balance may also require supplementing with potassium iodide. You'll need a prescription but this form of iodine can be a powerful push of a woman's physiology toward healing and health. Your doctor will request potassium iodide as SSKI.

The Power of the Mind

Millions of American women eat the standard American high-fat, low-fiber, vegetable-poor, protein-rich diet. Yet cervical cancer is far less common than the prevalence of herpes and genital warts would suggest. When analyzing risk factors for any kind of cancer, we must factor in the power of the mind.

One research project did just that, and found that women with cervical cancer tended to dislike sexual intercourse, had orgasm less often, had leukorrhea (vaginal discharge) more often, had a tendency to marry alcoholics, and a high incidence of divorce compared to women who developed cancer at other sites. In addition, women with cervical cancer more often came from a family in which a parent was absent or dead, and felt they had received inadequate love as a child.

Two other researchers predicted with significant success which women in a group biopsied because of abnormal Pap smears would have cancer and which would not, relying exclusively on the degree of hopelessness they seemed to exhibit, that is, women who felt they were the "cause" of all that had happened, yet believed they could do nothing to change their situation, who focused exclusively on caring for others and felt guilt or shame when their goals were not achieved. This psychological profile has been confirmed by other research studies.[4] Looking at the whole picture, we can profile a woman who felt an enormous need for love and looked for it through sexual relationships with men at an early age, who had a series of unfulfilling relationships, became infected with diseases that contributed to abnormalities of her cervical tissues, who gives up with a sense of resignation when relationships continually are unsatisfactory and losses recur, and who develops cancer when other contributing factors push her immune system over the brink.

Preventing Cancer

Body and mind work as a team, whether or not we are aware of this teamwork. Supplements are an important part of the cancer prevention program, yet the many factors that contribute to creating disease include environmental toxins, emotional distress, nutritional deficiencies, and the individual's perception of her ability to transform dysfunctional and unhealthy aspects of her life into factors that will support and enhance her health. It's a health package, and each woman creates it anew for herself, according to her life history and her current needs.

UTERUS
Uterine Cancer

Uterine cancer, also called endometrial cancer, is most often found in women past age 65, though it has occurred in younger women. Some of the risk factors that seem to be associated with this location of the disease are diabetes, obesity, having no children, having had breast cancer, and having excess estrogens circulating in the body.

In the chapter on menopause we discuss the rise in endometrial cancer resulting from the use of replacement estrogen for postmenopausal women. Younger women using sequential oral contraceptive pills are also at higher risk for this disease. Body fat converts androstenedione, an androgenic steroid from the adrenal glands, to estrone, a form of estrogen, so the more body fat a woman has, the more estrone is created. Consequently, obese women are more at risk of developing the two diseases associated with excess estrogen: breast cancer and endometrial cancer. Diabetes mellitus, early start of menstruation, and hypertension have also been associated with this form of cancer, in at least one one study.[5]

Since obesity is frequently tied in to feelings of low self-esteem, depression, anger, and self-destructiveness, there's always more to losing weight and reducing cancer risk than simply plunging into a diet. In addition, stress affects androstenedione production, so a reduction in cancer risk involves a deep look at the life one is living, and one's attitude toward what is going on in one's life.

Diet, Again

One study specifically looked at nutrition and diet in relation to endometrial cancer, comparing the diets of 206 patients suffering from endometrial cancer with 206 patients suffering from serious but noncancerous conditions. They discovered that a significantly greater number of women with endometrial cancer consumed more fat (as margarine, butter, and oil) and fewer green vegetables, fruit, and whole grain foods. The researchers concluded that endometrial cancer appears inversely related to the quantity of beta carotene and fiber consumed. In addition, they found that the woman with cancer consumed less milk, liver, and fish, but the same quantity of carrots, meat, eggs, and cheese as the controls.

In Finland, women with cancer of the ovary, uterus, or vulva were found lacking in selenium and the selenium-dependent enzyme glutathione peroxidase in their blood. Researchers at the University of Oulu gave both selenium and vitamin E supplements to these patients before initiating chemotherapy treatment. The combination of these two nutrients effectively lowered circulating peroxides in the cancer patients. Concentrations of peroxides are high in cancerous tissue and continue to be produced as cancer progresses, so the results of supplementation were considered beneficial in protecting the women's bodies from further damage.

In patients undergoing therapy for a variety of cancers, including uterine cancer, vitamin A and D levels were found to be low even before therapy began. After radiation therapy, levels of vitamin B-12, C, and E also dropped. Folic acid levels dropped significantly after either radiation or chemotherapy.[6] Please see our discussion of the benefits of taking supplements such as these during treatment with radiation or chemotherapy in the section on breast cancer in Chapter 1. We describe there how these nutrients not only replace those destroyed by the toxic treatments, but serve to minimize or prevent unpleasant side effects that frequently accompany these treatments, including hair loss.

Another supplement that may be needed by women who develop uterine cancer is iodine. Bruce V. Stadel of the Contraceptive Evaluation Branch, Center for Population Research, National Institute of Child Health and Human Development in Bethesda, Maryland, has documented the clear correlation between rates of breast, endometrial, and ovarian cancer and geographical location. Plotting cancer cases on a map reveals that incidence of these gynecological cancers is inversely correlated with dietary iodine intake, that is, these kinds of cancers occur most frequently in areas of low iodine availability. Women who develop these cancers eat fewer iodine-containing foods than women who don't have these cancers. Stadel hypothesizes that low dietary intake of iodine may produce borderline hypothyroidism. Low thyroid, even "normal" levels at the lower end of the scale, increases the production of estrogens by the ovaries, which overstimulates the growth of both breast and endometrial tissues (the endometrium is the inner lining of the uterus).

Take potassium iodide as a supplement, or increase iodine-rich foods, such as seaweeds and fish, and use kelp or dulse powder as a salt substitute. This provides the benefits of iodine in addition to useful minerals, without the additives in commercial iodized salt.

OVARIES

Ovarian Cancer

International health statistics indicate that cancer of the ovary is more common in Europe and North America than in Asia or Africa. Epidemiologists investigating this phenomenon have discovered a strong association between diet and cancer: Women who eat more fat have a higher incidence of ovarian cancer than women who eat a low-fat diet. In one study, carried out from 1957 to 1965, 274 women with a history of ovarian cancer were compared with 1,034 women having nonmalignant conditions. The researchers found that ovarian cancer risk decreased with increasing numbers of pregnancies. They could not find a relationship between ovarian cancer risk and cigarette smoking, frank thyroid disease, diabetes, or marital status, but ovarian cancer did seem to be associated with first marrying at a late age; being previously hospitalized for benign breast disease; and eating less vitamin A-rich foods (particularly in the 30–49 age group).

These results support other studies that connect cancer risk to endocrine and sex hormone imbalances and dietary deficiencies of vitamin A and its precursor, beta carotene.

Interestingly, the use of oral contraceptives seems to decrease the risk of ovarian cancer. Other complications of oral contraceptives, however, are serious enough, in our opinion, to offset this possible benefit. (See Chapter 6, on contraception, for more details.)

The fact that ovarian cancer represents only 15 to 20 percent of gynecological cancers, yet causes a disproportionate number of deaths, is attributable to the fact that ovarian cancer has no symptoms and advances without the woman's being aware of its presence. Preventive measures for ovarian cancer are similar to those for the other gynecological cancers:

- Lower fat intake and increase consumption of green and orange vegetables, fresh fruits, nuts, seeds, seafood, and whole grains.
- Add supplemental vitamins and minerals to the diet, particularly vitamins A, C, and E and the mineral selenium.
- Check for low thyroid and correct the hormone balance if necessary.
- Resolve stressful relationships.
- Release feelings of anger, resentment, and guilt and transform these strong emotions into positive affirmations of self-worth, self-confidence, and self-approval.

Ovarian Cysts

A cyst is a fluid-filled sac. Often, ovarian cysts are small and do not cause functional problems; sometimes they appear and then disappear within a couple of months. Cysts may interfere with ovarian function, however, contributing to a lack of menstruation and infertility. This more serious condition is called polycystic ovarian disease or Stein-Leventhal Syndrome.

Polycystic ovarian disease can be diagnosed from an examination—revealing enlarged ovaries in about half the cases—and a medical history: Often, the women began menstruating normally in adolescence, but over time their menstrual periods stopped coming. Frequently, sufferers are obese. About 50 percent of sufferers have unusually profuse body hair. These factors indicate a hormonal involvement with the condition.

The Thyroid Connection

According to Dr. Broda Barnes, one of the country's foremost authorities on thyroid hormone and health, women with ovarian cysts commonly suffer from low thyroid hormone. Barnes claims that correcting the underlying thyroid deficiency will often eliminate the cysts.[7] (See page 35 for details on self-testing of thyroid levels).

Why thyroid? Two reasons: Thyroid hormone prevents excess blood clotting (blood clotting promotes inflammation); it also helps speed the liver's detoxification of excess estrogen in the bloodstream.

A Cyst as a Defense Strategy

A cyst is one of the body's defense mechanisms. It can result from the body's failure to reabsorb the fluid of a partially developed hair follicle; or it may be a wall around toxic material that otherwise would poison surrounding tissues. This material might come from residues of cell metabolism, of a battle waged between the immune system and pathogenic organisms, or from poisons that the body cannot eliminate through normal channels and that therefore are carefully isolated until a future time, when the body will be able to cleanse itself of the watery irritants. We must look beyond the cysts themselves to their cause—a toxic body.

We recommend that anyone with cysts, be they on an ovary, the skin, or on any internal organ, immediately clean up her diet. Drink only pure, filtered water, never tap water. Eat organic produce if you can find it in farmer's markets or health-food stores. Eliminate sugar, coffee, black tea, soda pop, white flour, salt, dairy products, and any refined foods from your diet. Eat fresh fruits, vegetables (especially green and orange ones), whole grains, nuts, seeds, and sprouts. Purchase a couple of natural foods or vegetarian cookbooks and discover the delicious alternative of homemade, healthy foods. If you crave cold drinks, combine soda water with different juices and herbal teas for a much cheaper version of bottled "sparklers." If you crave dairy products, taste sweetened soy milk, or blend a half cup of almonds in three cups of water in your electric blender until the water turns white. Strain, saving the pulp for use in baking or cooking and drink the almond milk instead of cow's milk. In health food stores, purchase a variety of flavors of ice cream alternatives made with soy (Ice Bean, from The Farm Foods in Summertown, Tennessee) or rice (Rice Dream from Imagine Foods of Palo Alto, California).

The purpose of these possibly radical changes in your eating habits is the reduction in dietary fat and toxins and the increase in health-giving vitamins and minerals.

In addition, we recommend vigorous, regular exercise to help the body eliminate toxins through the skin via the sweat glands. And don't forget to drink enough water each day. Urination is another way to eliminate toxins, and cyst prevention and care includes the elimination of toxins as well as the prevention of toxic accumulations in your body. When the body's own immune system isn't overwhelmed, it can do the job of eliminating unwanted materials that may, if allowed to build up, contribute to the formation of ovarian cysts.

Supplements for Cysts

In addition to adequate thyroid hormone, a woman with ovarian cysts may want to consider taking supplemental Vitamin E and Vitamin B complex. Vitamin E has been found very useful for breast cysts (see Chapter One), and clinical experience indicates that the substance is equally beneficial in eliminating cysts on the ovary. Vitamin B Complex includes lipotrophic factors such as choline and inositol, which help the liver's detoxification of excess estrogen in the bloodstream. This helps prevent and eliminate ovarian cysts.

Daily Supplement Dose Advisory—Uterus and Ovaries

CERVIX

Cervical Dysplasia
  Folic acid—5 mg (this is unusually high, but we have found it therapeutic)
  B complex (or brewer's yeast)—50 to 100 mg of the major B vitamins
  Vitamin A—10,000 I.U.
  Vitamin C—at least 5,000 mg
  Vitamin E—800 I.U.
  Multimineral—look for trace minerals such as vanadium and molybdenum in the formula
  Potassium iodide—½ dropperful three times a day in a glass of water

Cervical Cancer
  Folic acid—5 mg
  Vitamin A—10,000 I.U.
  Vitamin C—to bowel tolerance
  Vitamin E—800 I.U.
  Selenium—200 mcg
  Potassium iodide—½ dropperful three times a day in glass of water

Uterine Cancer
Vitamin A—10,000 I.U.
Vitamin C—to bowel tolerance
Vitamin E—800 I.U.
Selenium—200 mcg
Multivitamin—a national brand purchased in a health-food store, not a drugstore house brand
Multimineral—One including trace elements such as manganese and vanadium

OVARIES

Ovarian Cysts
Vitamin E—800 I.U.
B complex—50 to 100 mg of the major B vitamins
Thyroid—(prescribed by doctor)
(or thyroid glandular)—take as directed on label

Ovarian Cancer
Vitamin A—10,000 I.U.
Vitamin C—to bowel tolerance, starting with 5,000 mg
Vitamin E—800 I.U.
Selenium—200 mcg
Multivitamin—a national brand at health-food stores, not drugstore house brand
Multimineral—look for trace minerals such as vanadium, molybdenum in formula

Chapter Three:

Vagina

In Brief—Vagina

VAGINAL CANCER

Symptoms—Bleeding or bloody discharge.

Signs—Laboratory testing of sample of vaginal cells confirms diagnosis.

Cause—Toxicity, hormonal imbalance.

Due to—Unknown cause or DES exposure in utero, coupled with depressed immune function.

Solution—Change diet; recognize and work through toxic thoughts and attitudes; take supplements, in addition to treatment agreed upon by oncologist and patient.

Supplements—Vitamins A, C, and E; selenium; multivitamin; multimineral.

VAGINITIS

Symptoms—Foul-smelling discharge.

Signs—Laboratory analysis reveals pathogenic agent.

Cause—Bacteria or virus coupled with abnormal vaginal pH and depressed immune system.

Due to—Improper diet, emotional stress, exposure through intercourse with infected partner.

Solution—Change diet; use herbal douches; take supplements; treat infected partner; improve personal hygiene; strengthen immune system with regular exercise, nutritious food, rest, stress reduction.

Supplements—Vitamin C, multivitamin, zinc, iron, caprylic acid, lactobacillus, potassium iodide.

GENITAL HERPES

Symptoms—Tingling or itchy feeling at specific site on skin of penis, buttocks, or vagina, followed by eruption of a cluster of small, blistery red bumps which last anywhere from a few days to several weeks.

Signs—Laboratory analysis of fluid within herpes lesion confirms diagnosis of this viral infection.
Cause—Exposure to infection through skin-to-skin contact, coupled with reduced efficiency of immune system and lowered resistance to infection.
Due to—Improper diet, nutritional deficiencies, emotional stress, physical trauma (as in abrasive intercourse, rape).
Solution—Improve diet, adjust diet to state of health, take supplements, reduce emotional stress, increase mental and physical exercise.
Supplements—Lysine, brewer's yeast or B complex, bioflavonoids (especially quercetin), vitamin E, vitamin C, vitamin A, zinc, B-12, BHT.

VAGINAL CANCER

We mention vaginal cancer in spite of its rarity because about six million women between 1943 and 1970 were given diethylstilbestrol (DES) as a miscarriage preventive and for other medical reasons. Only in the last 15 years or so has the ordinary clinician been forced to recognize the clear connection between this unnecessary drug and vaginal cancer in the daughters of women who received it. Suddenly, a disease that was once limited to women over 70 is appearing in very young women, even teenagers.

In the case of vaginal cancer our advice is the same as that for any gynecological cancer, so we suggest you read the sections on breast cancer in Chapter 1 for our suggestions on changing diet, attitude, and life-style to prevent cancer, stimulate the immune system to rid the body of cancer, and minimize the damage of radiation and chemotherapy treatments.

VAGINITIS

The suffix "itis" refers to an inflammation. It implies swelling, redness, and pain. Vaginitis is a very common problem. It usually isn't serious or permanently damaging, but it can be, so it's important to take care of any form of vaginitis promptly.

A white or clear mucous discharge is a normal part of the body's self-cleansing system. The quantity, odor, and other characteristics of this healthy discharge vary from woman to woman, except during her fertile days, when each woman's discharge changes from opaque to clear and from sticky to stringy, just like the consistency of egg whites, which is a convenient signal flag for those concerned about avoiding or creating a pregnancy. Though odor is a personal sensation, the scent of a healthy vaginal discharge is not unpleasant.

If you notice a strong, unpleasant odor or see a white cheesy discharge, or a greenish-colored one, and have itching, painful urination, or painful intercourse, you probably have a vaginal infection.

There are many different kinds of infection of the vagina, including bacterial *(Hemophilus* or *Chlamydia),* fungal (yeast), parasitic *(Trichomonas),* and viral (herpes). We are not going to discuss all of them in detail, but we'll sketch the broad outline of their development and elimination, and focus on what's most important in relation to supplements.

When discussing vaginal infections, it's important to remember that bacteria and viruses exist in your body starting a few hours after birth. Most of the microorganisms that live inside your vagina are harmless, and since many compete for the same nutrients, they help keep each other in check. It is only when your resistance is lowered, or the normal balance of organisms is altered, that certain of the organisms multiply beyond control and cause vaginitis.

You must also be aware that men harbor these organisms in their urethras or beneath their foreskins, and they can reinfect you after you clear yourself of an infection. This is avoided by treating your partner when you are treated and being more careful about personal cleanliness before, during, and after intercourse.

One of the most serious consequences of vaginitis occurs when the infection is untreated and moves up the vagina into other areas, causing pelvic inflammatory disease (PID). This can lead to chronic pain and internal scarring that interferes with the normal functioning of the reproductive organs. Infertility is a common result of PID, so beware and be wise: Take care of any abnormal vaginal discharge promptly.

Postmenopausal Vaginitis

In women past menopause, or in younger women whose ovaries have been removed surgically, irritation of the vagina may occur without the infection of a microorganism.

The vaginitis of the postmenopausal (or surgical menopausal) patient is easiest to treat. Look on page 157 in the chapter on menopause for details.

Preventing Vaginitis

If you are frequently bothered by vaginal infections, it's time for an inventory of your habits, clothes, relationships, and food. Your body is clearly protesting the way you are creating your life.

First of all, you must have a strong immune system to keep belligerent organisms in their place. Your resistance to infection—any infection—is based on regular exercise, nutritious food, clean water, sufficient rest, effective stress reduction, and personal hygiene. We are talking about daily habits, not occasional binges of taking good care of yourself. Eating some vegetables a few times a week isn't enough to keep your immune system functioning at its optimum. Neither is a once-a-month bike ride with friends, or sleeping late on weekends after going nonstop all week.

Down to Specifics: Personal Hygiene

Personal hygiene isn't taught to everyone, though many women are counseled in such matters by their mothers. If you never were advised on this subject, here's a rundown on the procedures that are crucial for your vaginal health:

· Wipe from front to back after a bowel movement, to prevent fecal material from coming in contact with your vaginal lips.
· Urinate after sexual intercourse, to wash away germs that may be lurking around the opening of your vagina.
· Avoid deodorant tampons, deodorant sanitary napkins, scented douches, scented toilet paper, or any product containing chemicals that comes in contact with your vagina, as it may cause irritation. Douching is of benefit only to the companies who sell the products. Women never need to douche, except as a medical treatment. If your vaginal secretions smell or taste unpleasant, you most likely have an infection. Otherwise, the secretions are useful and needed by your body for lubrication and the elimination of cellular waste.
· Wear cotton underpants, or, the very least, panties with a cotton crotch. Cotton absorbs sweat. Nylon and artificial materials force the sweat to remain against the body, creating ideal conditions for the development of yeast: warmth, moisture, and nutrients in vaginal secretions.
· Sleep without underwear. If you are bothered by infections, go without underwear while working in the kitchen or around the house, to allow optimum air circulation to your vagina.

Treating Vaginitis

Popping a pill and considering it adequate treatment for a vaginal infection is about as useful as wiping the kitchen counter once with Lysol and considering that a permanent solution to a dirty kitchen. Medicine may be part of the solution, but the cure is a result of changes in your life, not a few milligrams of a bactericide.

In fact, vaginitis medication may be dangerous to your health! Flagyl (G.D. Searle & Company's trade name for the drug metronidazole) has been linked in animal studies to cancer, birth defects, and genetic mutations. After several years of pressure from public-interest health organizations, The Food and Drug Administration forced the manufacturer to change the label in 1976 to indicate the possibility of human carcinogenicity and to recommend a lower dose of the drug. Nevertheless, metronidazole has consistently been the treatment of choice for a parasitic infection called trichomonas as well as the bacterial infection called either Hemophilus vaginalis or Gardnerella, and is still the most successful agent used by physicians to counter these infections. The FDA concluded that the benefits of the medicine outweigh its risks. We feel it is especially important that you complement this drug treatment with immune system–enhancing practices and nutrients.

One of the most important self-care treatments for vaginitis is to change your vaginal pH. The influence of pH on health is one of the most under-recognized factors in considering why certain people become ill and in treating any disease with natural methods. On the pH scale, 7 is neutral. Below 7 is increasing acidity. Above 7 is increasing alkalinity. The change in pH created by food and drink is one of the factors that allows us to manipulate our health with our fork and spoon. In the case of the vagina, microorganisms that are kept in check by an acidic pH can flourish in a more alkaline environment. For example, both Trichomonas parasites and Gardnerella bacteria happily multiply at a pH of 5 to 5.5. A healthy vagina is more acidic, from 3.8 to 4.2 on the pH scale.

Here is a list of alternatives to drug therapy (if you are pregnant, for example, or just want to try nontoxic approaches first) and supplemental treatments you can use in addition to drugs. Don't forget to add our personal hygiene suggestions to these suggestions. You can use these treatments even if you are menstruating. But be sure to be tested for venereal disease and pelvic inflammatory disease before undertaking self-treatment.

· Vitamin C to bowel tolerance. Take enough to cause loose stools, then reduce dosage until stools are firm again. As you heal, your body will need less and less vitamin C; the amount your body needs can be reliably adjusted according to bowel tolerance.
· Vitamin A—Always useful for healing from infections of any kind. We especially recommend the vitamin's precursor, beta carotene, which is an effective infection fighter and, unlike vitamin A, is *not* toxic even in high doses.
· Vitamin E—Helps vitamin A, and is a good healing agent on its own.
· Zinc—Also an effective healing agent. Actually speeds the healing of injured tissues.
· Iron—Deficiency sets you up for chronic vaginitis.
· B complex or brewer's yeast—Useful for helping you relieve stressful feelings, harmonizing the nervous system, helping regulate the sex hormones. In the case of herpes, helps lysine be absorbed better.
· L-lysine—The premier amino acid for preventing and treating a herpes attack.
· Cranberry juice—This will help acidify your system. Drink only a brand from the health-food store without added sugar. It may be mixed with another juice to sweeten it.
· Hot sitzbath—The purpose of this sitzbath is to increase the temperature of your genital area only, to stimulate blood circulation and promote healing. Let a few inches of very hot water into the bathtub, and sit in it with your hands and feet propped up out of the water.

With any of the following douches, you may use a regular douche bag, or you may place the active ingredients in a small amount of warm bath water, and with your fingers spread your vaginal lips to allow the fluid to wash in and out of the vagina. This is an alternative to actually douching with a douche bag. If you use such a bag, be sure to allow the fluid to gush out first, rather than sticking the tube inside and forcing whatever air is in the tube into your vagina ahead of the medicinal fluid. Instead of a douche bag, you can purchase an infant syringe, which has a conveniently long spout attached to a rubber bulb. Run hot water in the tub just to warm it up, or allow the shower to beat down on the tub for a few moments. Lie down with your knees up in the empty, now-warm tub. Take the douche solution into the tub with you in a jar or plastic container, and transfer the fluid to your vagina using the syringe. Stay horizontal for a while, to keep the fluid inside as long as possible.

Betadine douche—2 tablespoons in 1 quart of warm water. Available from pharmacies. Beware—it stains, so use it in the bathtub and rinse both yourself and the tub well.

Vinegar douche—1 teaspoon in 1 quart of warm water at bedtime. Use only once a day, as vinegar can dry out mucous membranes. Vinegar restores the acidic environment normal to a healthy vagina.

Acidophilus is the organism that usually keeps the infective agents in your vagina in line. When you take a course of antibiotics, or when the vaginal pH changes, these "good guys" are killed or their numbers are diminished and the "baddies" overwhelm the area. By reintroducing cultures of acidophilus, you can rebalance the microorganism menagerie and restore peace within. Some women use plain yogurt as a douche. Make sure it is Continental, Alta Dena, or a health-food store brand that contains live acidophilus cultures—never use the sugary kind with fruit added. At a health-food store you can also purchase the acidophilus culture itself as a liquid. Keep it refrigerated.

Yogurt and lemon juice douche—combines the helpful lactobacillus organisms with the acidity of the lemon juice. Squeeze one lemon, strain, and add to a couple of tablespoons of plain yogurt. The cool yogurt soothes irritated tissues and minimizes the sting of the juice. To insert the mixture, lie back in a warmed bathtub with your feet against the wall or in the air. Open your vaginal lips with the fingers of one hand, and feed the mixture into your vagina with a spoon (keep the spoon in the bathroom for future use—don't return it to your kitchen drawer). The coolness of the metal spoon will feel good against itchy or sore tissues. Remain horizontal a few moments, to let the douche remain inside. Rinse off your crotch and use a sanitary pad on your underwear to catch drips for the next few hours.

Goldenseal—This herb is an excellent bacteria fighter, helping the immune system to eliminate infections of any kind. Cover 1 teaspoon of goldenseal with 1 quart of boiling water, and steep until cool. Strain. Use daily. You may want to add a clove of garlic to the goldenseal when you steep it, as garlic, too, can eliminate a number of organisms, including mycobacterium, bacteria, and the strains of yeast that cause vaginitis.[1] In health-food stores you can purchase liquid garlic capsules with the pungent odor removed.

Plain old ordinary baking soda—Also an effective douche solution, though this seems contrary to our other advice, since the soda is alkaline. It may be that microorganisms cannot exist in an environment that is too acidic or too alkaline—they need a narrow range of values to prosper. Use about 2 teaspoons to a quart of water.

Potassium sorbate—A preservative you may be avoiding in packaged foods and beverages, it is used by manufacturers to retard yeast growth and extend the shelf life of their products. It also retards the growth of yeast in your vagina. A pharmacy can provide you with potassium sorbate in a concentrated stock solution. We are not fans of preservatives in any body orifice, but add this treatment to your list of yeast-fighting weapons.

Nutritional Self-Defense

Whatever strengthens the immune system will help you return your vagina to health. A diet heavy on acidic foods, including beans and grains, is a special focus for the week or weeks you're working on curing vaginitis. And eliminate any sugar, white flour, and refined foods from your diet during this time. We hope you leave these unnutritious substances—we can't call them food— for rare times during holidays or special celebrations, rather than including them in your daily menus.

You will want to up your intake of vitamin A–rich foods, the orange fruits and vegetables and dark-green leafy vegetables. And you will want to drink much more water than you are probably used to consuming. Aim for eight glasses of water (filtered, please) a day, to help your body eliminate through urine and stool whatever toxic matter it can.

HERPES

Only a few years ago, the press flung the specter of herpes in the face of young Americans as though it were the plague. Some women and men were sure their sex lives were over once they received a diagnosis of this viral disease; for those not yet resigned to eternal celibacy, herpes dating services formed as if those with herpes needed to be isolated from the rest of society. Today, with HIV/AIDS as the new plague, women who only have herpes sigh with relief.

Once the public spotlight was off herpes, common sense could prevail. After all, no one formed dating services for those suffering from cold sores, chicken pox, or shingles, yet these are variant strains of the herpes virus.

No woman becomes distraught when, as regular as clockwork, she comes down with a winter cold. She may notice that during the winters when she is taking special care of herself, isn't run down, eats well, rests plenty, and is feeling happy with her relationships and her life, she doesn't have her usual sniffles. When she resumes her old bad habits, back to bed she goes with the familiar fever-cough-sneeze routine.

Herpes is like a common cold in that what you do between outbreaks has a lot to do with the existence, duration, and intensity of outbreaks. However, while a good sneeze can spread cold germs around a room, herpes is usually passed from person to person via intimate contact. That contact doesn't have to be sexual. Wrestlers get herpes from each other. However, women usually get the disease from an infected man during sexual activity.

Some people are afraid of catching herpes from toilet seats. One researcher found that herpes did live as long as four hours on toilet seats, but transfer of the infection by this route is unlikely, according to Maryanne Dillon, of the UCLA Division of Infectious Diseases. First, as the virus-filled fluid from the active herpes lesion dries on the seat, the herpes viruses die. Second, the skin of legs and buttocks is fairly tough and relatively impermeable to contagion, unlike the mucous membranes, which are the usual route of transmission. Third, contact with the material left on the seat wouldn't be prolonged, unlike that of intercourse, when the delicate skin of the penis and vagina rub with great friction for extended periods of time.

The Eruption

Small, blistery red bumps cluster on or around the vagina, or mouth or buttocks, after a tingling or itchy feeling of several hours or even a day or two that warns of the imminent eruption. The sores are filled with fluid, and are painful. Sitting can be uncomfortable. Within a few days scabs form. Eventually the scabs disappear, and the skin returns to normal. The process may last as long as three weeks, or as briefly as a few days. The very first eruption is usually the worst, with the added discomforts of swollen lymph glands, muscle aches, and fever.

There has been a great deal of publicity about the observed association between genital herpes and cervical cancer. However, no cause-effect relationship has been established. It could just as easily be a case of a deficient immune system allowing two separate invasive, pathogenic processes to occur simultaneously. Whether a woman has herpes or not, we advocate a yearly Pap smear for every woman as part of her regular self-care routine.

A proven serious complication of herpes is an outbreak during pregnancy. The Los Angeles chapter of HELP (See For Further Information), a herpes education and self-help organization, estimates that in Southern California, around 35 percent of deliveries in women with a history of herpes are cesarean sections because the mother has an active case of herpes at the time of delivery. A cesarean protects the infant from potential blindness resulting from contact with the virus on the way down the birth canal, if the surgery occurs before the waters break. A woman with herpes can deliver vaginally if cultures taken twice weekly after the thirty-sixth week of pregnancy remain negative. If the mother doesn't have active herpes lesions, the infection rate at birth is only 8 percent. However, if she has active lesions, the infection rate jumps to 50 percent and since mortality rates among untreated babies can be as high as 65 percent, herpes isn't something to forget to report to your midwife or obstetrician.

The Elusive Virus

Cold sores are herpes virus infections of the mouth and lips. The virus is virtually the same as the one that infects the genitals, but is called herpes simplex virus I (HSV I), in contrast to the genital variety, which is called herpes simplex virus II (HSV II). It has been estimated that 90 percent or more of the population has been exposed to herpes simplex virus I. About

25 percent of sexually active adults have had at least one outbreak of HSV II, and many more carry the antibody to the virus, indicating that they have been exposed, though they have never broken out with the infection. In a UCLA study of couples in which one partner had herpes, 25 percent of the partners who believed they were herpes-free actually had antibodies to the disease in their blood, indicating that they had been exposed and their bodies had reacted to the disease, even if no vesicles, or blisters, had formed on the skin surface.

The ancient Greeks knew the wily habits of this virus; the name herpes comes from the Greek word meaning "to creep." Once the initial infection erupts on the skin, the virus slinks along the nerves to the spinal cord, where it hides out in the nerve ganglia in a dormant state until conditions are ripe for its reappearance. Fever, pregnancy, menstruation, stress, lack of sleep, overwork, emotional distress, improper diet, or exposure to sunlight, wind, and cold can all encourage a new eruption. For some, the infection recurs with infuriating frequency, while for others years may pass between outbreaks.

According to Centers for Disease Control statistics, as many as 500,000 new cases of genital herpes occur each year. Once you have contracted the virus, however, the frequency with which it reappears is directly under your control. Your diet, emotional state, physical health, and supplement program can make all the difference between the virus's being a minor inconvenience and a major disruption of your life.

Preventing Herpes

The key to prevention of herpes transmission is not only being careful. *It's also important to realize that you may be asymptomatic and still be shedding herpes virus.* This is a new and disquieting finding. Even without manifesting any sign of the disease, one partner may be able to infect the other. This is not the same thing as having a lesion on your cervix which is so hidden that you might not feel it and most certainly won't see it. In such a case, a woman could transmit the virus to an unsuspecting partner. But new research also suggests that someone who does not have an active lesion anywhere on his or her body can still infect another. Daniel Skiles, president of the Los Angeles Chapter of HELP, advises, "Look for clear skin, but that may not be enough!" According to Skiles, the only really safe sex is in the context of a monogamous relationship with someone known and trusted.

Safe sex means using both a condom and spermicide when engaging in sexual intercourse, unless you are actively trying to get pregnant. The spermicide contains nonoxynol-9, which kills herpes virus on contact. The condom protects you from virus that may be being shed by your partner, and protects your partner from virus you may be shedding. Skiles points out that the condom covers only a limited amount of the total body surface that might be infected and shedding virus, since herpes simplex virus II may strike anywhere below the waist.

A man's anatomy being what it is, it's unlikely that he'll be unaware of herpes lesions on his penis or scrotum. Nevertheless, as a first line of protection, you must take the initiative and inspect your partner before you flip off the lights. At least one young woman of our acquaintance rues the day she assumed her new lover was healthy. She discovered too late that he had herpes scabs visible on his penis (which were rubbed off, of course, by the friction of intercourse). The woman refused to see him again, but carries a reminder of her lack of self-care to this day, since now she has herpes.

In contrast, there are couples who live together and don't pass the disease between them. How do they do it? First, they are concerned enough about each other's well-being to prevent passion and sentimentality from getting in the way of the extra time it takes to be careful. Second, there is some indication that exposure to shedding, in the absence of active lesions, creates a kind of vaccination effect, creating antibodies in the uninfected partner against the disease, but not challenging the immune system enough to break out in lesions.

What about oral sex? If you or your partner has active lesions, you must avoid contact of any sort. If you are afraid you might have a hidden lesion on your cervix, you may feel assured by the lack of any clinical evidence that herpes is easily passed from female cervix to male mouth. Practically speaking, the penis sustains far more contact with the cervix than a man's mouth ever can.

Avoiding Outbreaks

Although no serious studies of the role of stress in herpes outbreaks have been undertaken, many people recognize that their outbreaks occur when they are under stress. In fact, the Herpes Resource Center, a nonprofit educational service of the American Social Health Association, offers a cassette tape titled *The Management of Herpes—an Approach to Conditioned Resistance*, which is specifically geared to stress reduction (see For Further Information for contact information). Some women with herpes have resorted to yoga, biofeedback, psychological counseling, or meditation in order to create consistent stress-reduction habits in their lives. For some, it took herpes to force them to slow down and take care of this important variable in the health equation.

If you read the magazines sold in health-food stores and on newsstands, you are probably already familiar with the herpes diet: low in the amino acid arginine, high in the amino acid lysine. This diet is based on the work of Dr. Christopher Kagan of UCLA, which he published in 1974. The medical community isn't 100 percent sold on the lysine-herpes connection, however, so you may not find much encouragement or information on this self-treatment in your doctor's office.[2] Some medical professionals consider the use of diet for treating herpes an elaborate placebo. We're in the camp which points to research such as a 12-month double-blind crossover study of oral herpes in which those taking 1,000 mg of L-lysine a day reported fewer outbreaks and those taken off lysine supplementation showed a significant increase in outbreak frequency.[3] This research indicated that it was less the placebo effect and more the objective blood level of L-lysine which best correlated with a drop in lesion frequency. We also keep handy the grand-daddy research project that inspired so many others—the 1978 study by Dr. Richard S. Griffith, professor of medicine at the Indiana University School of Medicine, and two colleagues, including Dr. Kagan, in which a whopping 96 percent of the 45 patients in the study given L-lysine experienced no further herpes outbreaks. Some were followed for as long as three years, without adverse reaction to the amino acid supplement and without a single eruption of the virus.

Additional weight to the lysine camp arrived from research at the Mayo Clinic Department of Dermatology, where a double-blind crossover study revealed that L-lysine in daily doses of over 1,000 mg effectively reduced the number and severity of herpes infections. Low doses (624 mg) were not as effective.

Since individuals vary in their ability to absorb nutrients and in their dietary intake of any particular nutrient, the amount of L-lysine that will eliminate herpes from your life may be quite different from that used by your best friend. Usually, 500 mg a day will keep herpes at bay, with many times that needed to stop an eruption once it occurs. Those with active sores may need to take 1,000 mg three times a day to clear it up quickly. Most signifi-cantly, those feeling the tingling signs of imminent outbreak may be able to thwart the virus entirely by taking this same high dose for several days. "Patients trying to establish a maintenance control dose would 'break through' when the amount of lysine ingested was cut back too much," re-ports Dr. Griffith and his colleagues. "Maintenance dosage varied with the individual, but it became obvious that no recurrence occurred in virtually all of the patients on 500 mg or more per day."

L-lysine appears to suppress symptoms, but to not cure the disease, so it must be provided to the body before outbreaks threaten or occur. It is hypothesized that in the absence of adequate concentrations of lysine, cells are more susceptible to viral invasion. Thus, what you put in your mouth is as important a virus-fighting tool as anything else you do.

A brief run-down on the best diet for preventing herpes outbreaks follows. If you don't believe us about the diet connection, pay attention to the inci-dence of herpes in your circle of acquaintances during Christmas and Easter, when chocolate consumption rises!

What's to Eat?

Potatoes
Yogurt
Fish
Fresh vegetables
Meat
Poultry

Eggs
Brewer's yeast
Soybeans
Legumes
Kefir

What's to Avoid?

Chocolate
Cocoa
Carob
Commercial gelatin mixes like Jell-O
Brown rice
Oatmeal
Raisins
Sunflower and sesame seeds
Whole-wheat bread
Popcorn
Eggplant
Tomatoes
Green peppers
Mushrooms
Peanuts and peanut butter, cashews, pecans, almonds
Sugar
Coffee and caffeinated tea

There is a difference between occasionally eating brown rice and making it the staple of your daily diet. The foods listed on the second list are high in the amino acid arginine and are among those frequently consumed the most by health-conscious people. We encourage you to not eliminate all of these foods entirely but to deemphasize arginine-high foods. Some, for example, are higher in arginine than others. The arginine-lysine ratio of peanuts, for example, is 3:1 and that of chocolate is 2:1, so these may have to be rare treats, while some of the others are closer to 1:1. In contrast, the ratio of arginine to lysine in potatoes is 1:2, making this vegetable an excellent choice in a herpes-prevention diet. As you pay more attention to the diet-herpes connection, you will be able to judge for yourself what foods, in what frequencies of consumption, lead to outbreaks.

Supplements for Herpes

· L-lysine.
· Vitamin C as calcium ascorbate (a useful antiviral agent)—Sheldon C. Deal, a Tucson, Arizona, naturopath and chiropractor, recommends killing herpes virus with 20 grams of vitamin C taken daily for a month. The Centers for Disease Control in Atlanta, Georgia, found that vitamin C

(sodium ascorbate) totally inactivated herpes viruses within 48 hours in a test-tube study. In a double-blind human study of recurrent oral herpes, a 600 mg water-soluble bioflavonoid–ascorbic acid complex caused remission of symptoms when taken as soon as the initial tingling of imminent eruption was sensed.

· Bioflavonoids, especially quercetin, the best virus-fighter among the bioflavonoids.
· Vitamin A.
· B complex, especially vitamin B-12.
· Vitamin E.
· Zinc.[4]
· BHT (butylated hydroxytoluene), an antioxdant used to retard spoilage in many foods, has a surprising use as a herpes fighter. We're not great fans of chemical medicines but must admit that some patients have experienced extraordinary results after taking BHT on a regular basis. Research suggests not taking over 250 mg per day.

External Treatments

The Santa Cruz Women's Health Center publishes a well-documented herpes information pamphlet (see For Further Information) that includes a number of nonprescription remedies for the itching and pain of herpes attacks.

They remind us, for example, that the tannic acid in black tea is a natural anesthetic, and recommend placing black tea bags soaked in hot water on the affected area.

Individuals have come up with a number of remedies that worked for them, including applying honey, vitamin E, witch hazel, wheat germ oil (a potent source of vitamin E), baking soda, aloe vera, or eucalyptus oil on the sores to help them dry up and heal. Others have used acupuncture to stimulate the body's infection-fighting powers.

Dr. Wyman Sanders, a Santa Monica psychiatrist, differentiates between herpes complex—the tumultuous emotions and social withdrawal people create as a result of contracting the disease—and herpes simplex, the disease, itself. "Herpes complex is devastating," says Sanders, "herpes simplex is not." To the participants in his herpes simplex support groups, he has repeatedly emphasized that they can, with attention to self-care, get to a point where the disease is no more than a nuisance. Samuel R. Knox of the American Social Health Association, writing in *Medical Self-Care* magazine, concurs. People are heartbroken because they have been told they have an incurable disease, yet herpes is, he suggests, as curable as the common cold. "The immune system goes to work on both these viral infections and cures them. Both can recur, in which case the body simply cures them again." *The Helper,* the newsletter produced by HELP, reminds us, "Always remember that herpes, as disruptive as it can sometimes be, is only a small part of who you are." See the end of chapter for more information on HELP.

Daily Supplement Dose Advisory—Vagina

VAGINAL CANCER

Vitamin A—10,000 I.U.

Vitamin C—to bowel tolerance, beginning with 5000 mg in divided doses

Vitamin E—800 I.U.

Selenium—200 mcg

Multivitamin—a national brand at health-food store, not a drugstore house brand

Multimineral—look for trace minerals such as vanadium, molybdenum

VAGINITIS

Caprylic acid—obtain concentrated liquid form and dilute as directed on label

Vitamin A—10,000 I.U

Vitamin C—to bowel tolerance

Vitamin E—800 I.U.

Zinc (elemental)—50 mg

Iron—100 mg (we prefer iron bound with other substances such as vitamin C, zinc, copper or magnesium)

Lactobacillus—best to purchase a brand containing several strains of organisms and which is kept in the store refrigerator section. Take as directed on the label

Potassium iodide—use as a douche: 1 dropperful in ½ cup water

HERPES

Vitamin A—10,000 I.U.

Vitamin C—to bowel tolerance

Bioflavonoids—at least 500 mg (be sure the product includes quercetin)

Vitamin E—800 I.U.

Zinc (elemental)—50 mg

L-Lysine—500 to 1,000 mg for prevention and up to 3,000 for acute outbreaks

Vitamin B complex—100 mg of major B vitamins

Vitamin B-12—at least 1,000 mcg

BHT—250 mg

Chapter Four:
Urinary Tract

In Brief—Urinary Tract

Symptoms—Burning, painful urination; urgency, pain during intercourse; fever; chills; strong-smelling and cloudy urine; in the case of nongonococcal urethritis (NGU), no symptoms.

Signs—Laboratory findings of E. coli, Ureaplasma, or Chlamydia; in the case of interstitial cystitis, no pathogens are present, but minute hemorrhages are seen in the bladder wall.

Cause—Transfer of anal bacteria to urethra; suppressed immune system; exposure to infected sexual partner; in the case of interstitial cystitis, possible complications of a yeast infection, systemic viral infection, or food allergies.

Due to—Inattention to lovemaking hygiene, or wiping back-to-front after urinating or defecating; drinking too little water; failing to urinate after intercourse; improper diet, with excess sugar; estrogen excess resulting from oral contraceptives; synthetic material in underpants; changing menstrual tampons or napkins too infrequently; use of perfumed or deodorized personal products; irritation from spicy food, alcohol, and caffeine; excess stimulation from motorcycles, long bicycle trips, or a vibrator; low thyroid; allergy; mechanical obstruction of circulation resulting from prolapsed transverse colon or abnormal bladder position following childbirth; liver or bowel congestion, leading to excessively toxic blood and urine passing through kidneys; or, in the case of NGU, sexual transmission.

Solution—Cranberry juice and vitamin C to acidify urinary tract; potassium iodide as antiseptic; drinking at least eight glasses of water a day; urinating after intercourse; hot baths; heating pads on lower abdomen; stop wearing pantyhose; wear cotton-crotch underwear; hold off intercourse until fully lubricated; make sure man's penis is clean beneath his foreskin; make sure man's body doesn't touch anus, then vagina, during intercourse; use positions during intercourse that do not irritate urethra; switch birth control from the Pill to a barrier method such as condom, cervical cap, or diaphragm plus spermicide; eliminate white sugar from your diet; take supplements; avoid allergens; treat systemic infections such as yeast or virus.

Supplements—Vitamin C, vitamin B-6, zinc, thyroid (or potassium iodide), B complex, beta carotene, vitamin A.

According to orthodox medicine, there are six major reasons why a woman could experience painful urination, painful intercourse, an urgent need to urinate, or blood in her urine: bladder cancer and gonorrhea (neither of which will be discussed in this book), E. coli infection (simple urinary tract infection—UTI), Chlamydia or Ureaplasma infection (nongonococcal urethritis—NGU), or interstitial cystitis. However, as Ross Trattler, a Hawaii-based naturopathic physician, points out, "The mere presence of bacteria will not cause an infection. If this were so, then *everyone* would have thousands of infections, both inside the body and out. Bacteria are an ever-present part of life."[1]

Trattler goes so far as to state that "bacteria found in urinary tract infections are the *result* of disease, not its cause." With urinary tract infections, as with every other condition described in this book, we urge you to consider your entire way of life as you look for causes of and treatments for your complaint. None of the factors we discuss occurs in a vacuum, but in the context of poor dietary choices, deficiencies of specific nutrients, and chronic stress. You may also suffer from constipation and liver congestion, which overwork the kidneys as they are forced to eliminate especially concentrated toxic body fluids. Even physical trauma that has misaligned your spinal column and spinal musculature can contribute to reflex irritation, poor circulation of blood and lymph, and greater susceptibility to infection of the genitourinary tract.

Drugs used to combat the infection can actually make matters worse. For example, penicillin is used against gonorrhea, but it is useless against Chlamydia and Ureaplasma, the main causes of nongonococcal urethritis. The drug that has the power to kill the disease-bearing organisms also kills useful bacteria that peacefully inhabit your intestinal tract. When the useful bacteria are wiped out, yeast (Candida albicans and other strains) proliferate unchecked and yet another infection rages. In fact, your urinary tract infection may be a symptom of systemic yeast infection: Sometimes yeast organisms in the bowel proliferate to such an extent that they pierce the mucous membrane of the intestinal lining and travel through the bloodstream to the weakest organ system, where they cause severe reactions. For some women, that system is the urinary tract, and taking antibiotics against the infection is like pouring oil on a fire.

BACTERIAL URINARY TRACT INFECTIONS

The most common cause of a urinary tract infection is an invasion of the urethra, the tube leading from the bladder to outside the body, by E. coli bacteria. This often occurs when a woman's defense system is working at less than peak performance, permitting the bacteria to run wild. Such urinary tract infections are the most frequent kind of infection after the common cold, striking as many as one in every five women each year.

Although urinary tract infections are most common in sexually active women, a decrease in estrogen after menopause can lead to thinning of the tissues of the bladder and urethra, making them vulnerable to infection.

Whatever the cause, an untreated urinary tract infection can spread to the kidneys, leading to serious complications.

In the fall of 1987 Norwich Eaton Pharmaceuticals of Norwich, NY, sponsored a survey of 200 women between the ages of 14 and 65 who had had a urinary tract infection treated by a physician. Seventy percent of those interviewed were married, and 80 percent had at least one child. Not surprisingly, 43 percent stated that their infection returned after initial treatment. A urinary tract infection is a symptom of a deficient immune system, and unless that system is nourished and regenerated, infections of one sort or another will plague the woman forever.

The survey pointed out some misconceptions about the problem, on the part of both women and the medical authorities. For example, many women believed that their sex partner gave them the urinary tract infection. What probably happened was that during sex play, some part of their partner's body touched the women's anus, then her vagina, transferring her own E. coli bacteria from its home in the bowel to the new site. Or the women themselves, may have wiped back to front after urinating or defecating, transferring E. coli bacteria to the vagina by their own poor bathroom hygiene.

Not surprisingly, the medical consultants hired by the pharmaceutical company pooh-poohed the idea that cranberry juice or yogurt could have any beneficial effect on a urinary tract infection, while 30 percent of women surveyed cited these self-care treatments as useful. A study conducted by Dr. Anthony E. Sobota of the Department of Biologic Science, Ohio State University (Youngstown), found that 15 ounces of cranberry juice taken by mouth resulted in 80 percent inhibition of bacterial growth, and there were other measurable signs of successful therapy in 15 out of 22 subjects. For example, for as long as three hours after their cranberry cocktail, the subjects' urine revealed less clinging of bacteria to bladder and urinary tract cells.[2]

Caffeine, on the other hand, can exacerbate a urinary tract infection. Women who smoke, drink alcohol, and consume coffee may be asking for such an infection for several reasons. Caffeine is a diuretic, and important minerals such as sodium, potassium, and calcium are lost in the urine with more frequent urination. While doctors frequently advise women prone to urinary tract infections to drink more than the usual amount of water to help flush out the bacteria, coffee drinkers may deplete their bodies of fluid and cause secondary problems as a result.

Water, however, is an excellent preventive for urinary tract infections. One urologist told a patient, "If women drank more water, I'd be out of business." Another simple but important preventive is to urinate after intercourse. Because a woman's urethra is placed so close to both her vagina and her anus, it is easy for bacteria to lurk at the urethra opening. The flow of urine flushes out such bacteria, preventing an infection.

According to Dr. Richard A. Kunin of San Francisco, water with a few drops of potassium iodide in it is all some women need to eliminate their chronic urinary tract infections. Potassium iodide is sold under the trade name SSKI. Kunin, the author of *Mega-Nutrition* and *Mega-Nutrition for Women* (both New American Library, $3.95) and a past president of the Orthomolecular Medical Society, suggests four to ten drops of potassium iodide in a half glass of water taken three times a day, and claims that this old remedy, probably in use over 100 years ago, is simply too old-fashioned and too well known to be credited by modern physicians. It is, he says, "underappreciated and overlooked through both naive ignorance and arrogance" on the part of American physicians. Urinary tract infections may be the "scourge of modern women," but Kunin finds that potassium iodide makes eliminating the problem "look mighty easy." Potassium iodide is sold by prescription as an antiseptic and expectorant. It clears mucous from the body and heals infections. Kunin has, himself, found over 70 uses for the old remedy. We haven't discussed many drugs, but this one is fairly safe, though it is contraindicated for people who are hyperthyroid or sensitive to iodides. A possible side effect is gastrointestinal discomfort.

We mentioned estrogen deficiency as a contributing factor in these infections, but excess estrogen causes problems, too, and women on oral contraceptives are especially susceptible to urinary tract infections. Another hormonal imbalance that contributes to increased infections is low thyroid (see page 35 for an easy home test for low thyroid).

On the mechanical side, obstruction of circulation by a prolapsed transverse colon or abnormal bladder position following childbirth can also contribute to the development of urinary tract infections, as can mechanical irritation from a vibrator or motorcycle. Chemical irritation from perfumed, deodorized, or colored personal-care products such as tampons and douches is a notorious offender. Even spicy food, coffee, or alcohol may cause biochemical irritants in the urine of sensitive women.

No More UTIs

Once the causes of your persistent infections have been revealed, you can take charge and eliminate the problem by taking the following steps:

· Drink cranberry juice and take vitamin C, to acidify the urine and heal the infection.

- Drink at least eight glasses of water a day to flush out bacteria and dilute your urine.
- Urinate after intercourse.
- Take hot baths and use heating pads to draw more blood to the area and promote healing.
- Wear a garter belt and thigh-high nylon stockings instead of pantyhose; wear underpants with cotton crotches.
- Make sure you are fully lubricated before your partner enters you during sexual intercourse, to prevent chafing, and make sure he cleans beneath his foreskin before you begin sex play.
- Use positions during sex that don't irritate your urethra.
- Switch from birth control pills to a barrier method, such as a condom, cervical cap, or diaphragm plus spermicide.
- Eat a wholesome, immune system–strengthening diet of green, orange, and yellow vegetables, fresh fruits, whole grains, nuts, seeds, and seafoods. Eliminate white sugar and white flour products, and cut down on dairy foods (which are high in fat and calories, highly allergenic, and are healthy only for baby cows in the form of whole raw milk).
- Take supplements to help heal from a current infection and prevent recurrences.

Supplements for Urinary Tract Infections

Vitamin C and bioflavonoids are high on the list of supplements useful for treating a urinary tract infection, as are vitamin A and beta carotene. Zinc and vitamin A help the body heal injured, irritated tissues. There is some evidence that people low in vitamin B-6 are more susceptible to genito-urinary tract infections.[3]

NONGONOCOCCAL URETHRITIS

A woman may be suffering from an invasion of Chlamydia, a parasite, or Ureaplasma, a strange little bacterium without a cell wall that has the disquieting habit of changing forms. Infection by either of these is commonly called "nongonococcal urethritis." Chlamydia diagnosis necessitates a complicated laboratory procedure. Yet Chlamydia infection has replaced gonorrhea as the number one sexually transmitted disease in the United States. Even more people have NGU than herpes.

Unfortunately, a woman may have no symptoms whatsoever. If she's lucky, she'll have warning symptoms—an itching or burning sensation in her genital area, or a yellow-white odorless discharge and dull abdominal pain. She may bleed between menstrual periods. Since Chlamydia is so easy to miss, it all too frequently moves up the woman's genito-urinary tract to her Fallopian tubes and into the pelvis, causing pelvic inflammatory disease. The consequences are often either infertility or ectopic pregnancy (pregnancy located in the Fallopian tube instead of the uterus).

If a pregnant woman suffers from a Chlamydia infection, there is a risk of stillbirth or premature birth, and the infant may contract the disease from the mother, which would affect its eyes and lungs.

Chlamydia is treated with tetracycline or erythromycin, plus careful use of a condom by the woman's partner during intercourse for three to six months following treatment. And the male partner must be treated at the same time, to prevent his reinfecting the woman.

INTERSTITIAL CYSTITIS

In the healthy body, the bladder extends like a rubber balloon as urine fills up its approximately 12-ounce capacity. With interstitial cystitis, the bladder wall becomes inflamed and scar tissue develops. The wall stiffens and no longer expands adequately, and the sufferer must rush to the bathroom as many as 60 to 100 times a day. Pain above the pubic bone is constant and intense. Sleep is nearly impossible, leading to irritability and depression. Although most sufferers are over 30, at least a fourth are younger than this. Interstitial cystitis was once considered a rare affliction, but the number of current cases is estimated at between 200,000 and 500,000.

Information on the personal side of the disease comes from a 1987 survey of about 1,000 women diagnosed with the condition, paid for by the National Institutes of Health and undertaken for the University of Pennsylvania by the Washington D.C.–based Urban Institute. Researchers found that pain during sexual intercourse occurred for two thirds of the women, half couldn't ride in a car without pain, and about half couldn't work full time, owing to the unrelenting pain and the constant need to urinate.

Putting the disease into a holistic framework, it is interesting to note that the researchers also discovered 10 to 12 times more childhood bladder problems among interstitial cystitis sufferers than among the general population. Tragically, as many as a half of those now suffering from interstitial cystitis are still receiving no relief from any treatment offered to them.

Dr. Robert Giller, a New York City general practitioner and coauthor of *Medical Makeover* has seen the maddening symptoms of this disease diminish once his patients eliminated from their menus diet sodas and other foods to which they have unrecognized sensitivities. Food allergies create biochemical irritants, which makes sense in the light of the women's history of childhood bladder complaints. We are reminded of pediatrician Lendon Smith's discovery that his son's bedwetting was, in effect, the child's bladder "sneezing" in an allergic reaction to the milk given him at school. The bladders of women with interstitial cystitis may also be reacting to allergenic foods with pain, stiffness, tiny hemorrhages, and chronic inflammation.

Santa Monica physician-acupuncturist Luc de Schepper suggests that food allergies may be part of a larger problem, that of systemic Candida albicans infection. The bladder complaints of three patients in whom another physician diagnosed interstitial cystitis disappeared once the woman followed the Candida elimination diet and took the supplements de Schepper prescribed. "If you looked for yeast you wouldn't find anything but dead yeast in the bladder," de Schepper claims. "If you had chronic diarrhea, eventually the elimination of toxins through your intestines would irritate your anus; similarly, the bladder becomes irritated after eliminating yeast for an extended period of time," he explains. The claim of Dr. Philip Hanno of the University of Pennsylvania that "some substance in the urine that irritates the wall of the bladder" may be to blame would tend to support de Schepper's hypothesis.[4]

Santa Monica naturopathic physician Janet Zand noticed that several women patients with interstitial cystitis also have a systemic viral condition, such as Epstein-Barr, which also affects the immune system. Zand's patients have benefited from avoiding any food they are allergic to, and staying entirely away from coffee. "Coffee definitely exaggerates interstitial cystitis," says Zand. She has also found that homeopathic remedies (diluted natural substances that stimulate the body's self-healing) and herbs are "very effective" in countering this condition.

Naturopathic physician Ross Trattler, who has a practice on the Hawaiian island of Maui, emphasizes the usefulness of looking at the life-style of the interstitial cystitis patient: "What are they doing to themselves that a healthy person would get sick by doing?" he asks. His treatment includes reversing whatever life-style factors may be involved (such as stress, diet, and lack of exercise) and improving the general vitality of the pelvic organs by means of alternating hot and cold sitzbaths and spinal manipulation. Sitzbaths, claims Trattler, are "the most effective measure in removing pelvic congestion and inflammation."

It is easy to give yourself a sitzbath treatment. Obtain two tubs 12 to 14 inches deep, big enough to allow you to immerse your entire pubic and pelvic region. Fill one with very hot water and one with ice-cold water. Sit in the hot tub and place your feet in the cold tub. After three minutes, reverse tubs. Repeat this cycle three times. Then briskly dry off with a rough bath towel. The contrast of water temperatures stimulates blood circulation to these areas, which removes congestion, draws nutrients to the areas, and speeds healing.

Orthodox and Unorthodox Treatments for Interstitial Cystitis

Orthodox treatments include stretching the bladder by forcing in fluid to break up scar tissue, or instilling the drug DMSO (dimethyl sulfoxide) into the bladder. DMSO is sold as Rimso (R)-50, by Research Industries Corporation of Salt Lake City and is a prescription drug. We don't emphasize drugs in this book, but DMSO at least has no contraindications and causes no chemical dependency; the only side effect is a garliclike taste in the mouth. DMSO relaxes muscles, dilates blood vessels, stops pain, and diminishes inflammation. Although it doesn't cure the condition, it can offer months of relief from the pain and urgent need to urinate. It isn't a picnic to have it instilled, however, so you will probably want to have anesthesia such as a saddleblock—similar to what is given to women during childbirth—during insertion of the drug into your bladder.

In addition to DMSO, you may want to do any or all of the following:

· Obtain acupuncture treatments, which can reduce stress, help eliminate pain, and relax muscles, including those of the bladder.
· See a homeopath/herbalist for appropriate remedies (see For Further Information.)
· Take the Candida albicans questionnaire that Dr. William Crook has prepared, and which appears on page 29 in his book *The Yeast Connection*. If it looks as though Candida is part of your problem, follow the self-care program detailed in Crook's book. Take supplemental acidophilus and bifidobacteria (obtainable in health-food stores) to recolonize your intestinal tract with friendly bacteria needed for proper digestion and assimilation of nutrients.
· Strengthen your bladder wall with supplements that are known to improve the health of mucous membranes and tissues, such as vitamin A and beta carotene, zinc, and bioflavonoids. Take care with vitamin C, though, as the acidity of this important infection fighter may easily backfire on you and exacerbate your discomfort.
· Eliminate allergenic food and environmental factors that might be contributing to or even causing your distress. Or see a clinical ecologist (a doctor oriented to environmental allergies) who can help you diagnose your sensitivities.
· Don't believe you have an incurable condition. The fact that symptoms come and go for many people is a good indication that sometimes they do something right, and at other times something wrong, for their body's well-being. There is no incurable disease, there are only diseases your doctor doesn't know how to cure.
· Learn and practice a relaxation technique to reduce stress and calm your nervous system, using biofeedback, meditation, visualization, breathing exercises, yoga, or any other system offered in your community that attracts you. Two books that may help are *You Can Heal Your Life* by Louise Hay and *Creative Visualization* by Shakti Gawain.

Daily Supplement Dose Advisory—Urinary Tract Infections

Vitamin C—to bowel tolerance
Vitamin A—10,000 I.U.
Beta carotene—100 mg
Zinc—50 mg
Vitamin B complex—100 mg of all major B vitamins
Potassium iodide—½ dropperful three times a day in a glass of water
  (prescribed by doctor)

Chapter Five:

Menstruation

In Brief—Menstruation

ABSENT MENSES: AMENORRHEA

Symptoms—No monthly menstrual bleeding.

Signs—Pregnancy, low estrogen, low progesterone, low basal body temperature, low FSH or other hormonal abnormalities, tumor, imperforate hymen, among other signs.

Cause—Nutritional deficiency, anatomical malformation, congenital defect, illness, emotional distress, drug side effect.

Due to—Diet, genes, overtraining, underweight, medical intervention.

Solution—Gain weight, lighten training, improve nutrition, take supplements, reduce stress, improve coping skills.

Supplements—Vitamin B-6, vitamin B-12, folic acid, zinc, thyroid, B complex, calcium, magnesium.

IRREGULAR MENSES

Symptoms—Arrival, volume, or duration of menses varies monthly.

Signs—Same

Cause—Low thyroid, high stress, abnormal body mechanics, organ prolapse, deficient B vitamins, other vitamin-mineral imbalances, disease, altered environment, drugs.

Due to—Severe dieting, improper choice of food, trauma, lack of exercise, childbirth, genetic predisposition, infection, fibroids, cancer, endocrine gland disorder, anemia, travel, antibiotics, allergy, candidiasis.

Solution—Wholesome diet, spinal manipulation, abdominal exercise, supplements in correct balance, de-stress environment.

Supplements—Vitamin B complex, vitamin B-6, vitamin C, zinc, lecithin, L-tyrosine, thyroid glandular, kelp.

TOO PAINFUL: DYSMENORRHEA

Symptoms—Painful abdominal cramps, backache.

Signs—Sometimes large blood clots are passed.

Cause—Overproduction of prostaglandin F-2-alpha, altered hormone levels, stress, anxiety, congestion or poor circulation of blood, nutritional deficiencies, muscle spasms, fibroid tumors, endometriosis, anatomical abnormality.

Due to—Improper diet; calcium/magnesium deficiency; relationship problems; work, financial, or household pressures; lack of exercise; genetic predisposition; abortion or miscarriage; IUD.

Solution—Correct diet, supplements; counseling; exercise program, yoga, or stretching; stress reduction and relaxation program; physical manipulation therapy; change birth control method; acupuncture.

Supplements—Calcium, magnesium, EFA (safflower oil, evening primrose oil, linseed oil, borage oil, or black currant oil), vitamin E, vitamin B complex, vitamin B-6, zinc, vitamin C.

TOO MUCH: MENORRHAGIA

Symptoms—Profuse menstrual flow.

Signs—Need for double pads or more than 12 pads per period.

Cause—Deficiency of vitamin B complex, vitamin A, vitamin C, bioflavonoids, vitamin E, vitamin K, zinc, lipotrophics, thyroid hormone, calcium.

Due to—Diet, hereditary deficiency.

Solution—Supplements, nutrient-rich diet, acupuncture.

Supplements—Thyroid; kelp; L-tyrosine; vitamins E, B-6, B complex, A, and C; bioflavonoids; zinc, iron, calcium, and magnesium; EFA (safflower oil, evening primrose oil, linseed oil, borage oil, or black currant oil); lipotrophics.

PREMENSTRUAL SYNDROME (PMS)

Symptoms—Mood shifts, craving sweets, breast pain, bloating.

Signs—Differs for different symptom groups.

Anxiety—high estrogen, low progesterone.

Bloating—high aldosterone, low dopamine.

Cravings—low blood glucose.

Depression—low norepinephrine, low estrogen, high progesterone.

Cause—

Anxiety—diseased ovary, poor liver function, decreased intestinal clearance, inadequate production of progesterone.

Bloating—vitamin B-6 deficiency, excess refined sugar.

Cravings—decreased glycogen in the brain, refined sugar intake, excess insulin, excess salt intake.

Depression—vitamin B-6 deficiency, tyrosine deficiency.

Due to—
  Anxiety—unknown cause, obesity, strenuous exercise, hepatitis, alco-
    holism, fiber deficiency, magnesium deficiency, vitamin B-6 defi-
    ciency, excess vitamin E, excess animal fats, stress.
  Bloating—poor dietary habits, lack of exercise, stress, cigarette smok-
    ing.
  Cravings—deficiencies in magnesium, B-6, linoleic acid, vitamin C,
    niacinamide, fiber.
  Depression—excess lead, vitamin B-6 deficiency, relative excess of
    male hormones (androgens).
Solution—
  Anxiety—supplements, diet change (cut caffeine; limit dairy, animal
    fat, and animal protein; increase vegetable protein, vegetable fat,
    fiber and complex carbohydrates); exercise; acupuncture.
  Bloating—supplements, exercise, reduce stress, moderate use of salt,
    limit simple carbohydrates, stop smoking cigarettes; acupuncture.
  Cravings—supplements, diet change—increase complex carbohy-
    drates; limit animal fats, dairy, salt, and simple carbohydrates such
    as pastries and other foods made with white flour and white sugar;
    avoid frequent snacks; acupuncture.
  Depression—supplements, lead detoxification, estrogen replacement;
    acupuncture.
Supplements—
  Anxiety—vitamin B-6, magnesium, riboflavin, B complex.
  Bloating—magnesium, vitamin B-6, iron, vitamin A, zinc, vitamin E.
  Cravings—magnesium, linoleic acid (safflower oil, evening primrose
    oil, linseed oil, borage oil, or black currant oil), chromium.
  Depression—same as for anxiety, plus tyrosine (morning) and trypto-
    phan (bedtime).

ABSENT MENSES—AMENORRHEA

There are times in a woman's life when the lack of menstruation, or amenorrhea, is normal: before puberty, during pregnancy, while nursing a baby, and
after menopause. Occasionally, a woman lacking periods is pleased by her
situation: a marathon runner who enjoys not having the hassle of periods
while competing, or a woman who does not want children, and enjoys her
lack of periods as a hassle-free form of birth control.

Menstruation, however, is the expression of a healthy body. It is a result
of a complicated orchestration involving two sections of the brain, the hypothalamus and the pituitary gland; two organs, the ovaries and the uterus; and
a precise counterpoint of hormones, including follicle-stimulating hormone
(FSH), luteinizing hormone (LH), estrogen, and progesterone. Amenorrhea
means some part of the orchestra is out of key.

One of the long-term effects of amenorrhea is osteoporosis, the "brittle bones" that are usually associated with old age, since lack of estrogen in even a young woman will permit mineral loss to occur. Although there are times when a woman ovulates but does not menstruate, such as may occur during lactation, for the most part amenorrhea signals infertility. Occasionally, it may be a sign of a tumor in the pituitary or adrenal glands or the ovary, which has its own dangers.

What to do about amenorrhea depends, of course, on the cause of the problem. It may be caused by malfunctioning glands, or result from malnutrition (including deficiencies of vitamin B-6 and zinc), obesity—or the opposite, too little body fat. It may occur in women marathoners or dancers who train too hard. It could also be due to metabolic problems, such as diabetes, liver disease, or abnormally low or high thyroid hormone levels. It can result from emotional distress. And it may be caused by certain drugs, such as morphine, nitroglycerin, or thallium (a radionuclide), or be a temporary effect of stopping birth control pills. Radiation of the uterus or ovaries and "surgical menopause"—hysterectomy—are other causes. Amenorrhea may also be a result of lead or mercury poisoning, fever, or severe anemia. Women's menstrual cycles represent a delicate interplay of emotions, environment, and anatomy. Even travel or extreme changes in a woman's surroundings can prevent a normal cycle. In a woman who has never had intercourse, amenorrhea may result from a lack of a small opening in the hymen, the membrane that stretches across the vaginal opening.

Primary amenorrhea is when menstruation fails to begin before the age of 16. If menstruation has occurred, but after a number of years stops, then it is called secondary amenorrhea.

Whether yours is primary or secondary, if you cannot isolate one of the more obvious causes, and a medical examination has ruled out pregnancy, tumors, and chronic disease, it's time to begin a hormone balancing act through your diet and life-style.

In a healthy woman, each month the front lobe of the pituitary secretes two hormones, follicle-stimulating hormone (FSH) and luteinizing hormone (LH). The FSH is released first, and chemically stimulates the ovaries into secreting estrogen, which in turn alerts the uterine lining to begin building up a good blood supply. The luteinizing hormone also stimulates the uterine lining, as does progesterone, another hormone secreted by the ovaries.

After an egg bursts through the wall of the ovary, the site of the "wound" in the ovary wall becomes a specialized gland, called the corpus luteum, which secretes more progesterone. Progesterone from the corpus luteum takes over the major role of developing a rich blood supply along the walls of the uterus, in preparation for possible implantation of an egg. If no egg implants in the uterus, the corpus luteum stops secreting progesterone, and the ovary slows down its estrogen supply. This drop in both estrogen and progesterone levels allows the unneeded blood along the uterine wall to be sloughed off as the menstrual flow. Clearly, progesterone levels must rise and then fall for proper menstruation to occur.

Amenorrhea may result from too little or too much hormone. In the middle of one patient's senior year in high school, her mother took her to the gynecologist to find out why she hadn't started menstruating yet. The teenager herself was happy to be avoiding all the mess and pain she saw her friends going through each month, and complained to her diary that she didn't see why everyone was so eager to nudge nature along. But she accepted the monthly hormone injection that brought on menstruation, until she went away to college in the fall.

The physician did not check this girl's body's supply of vitamin B-6 and zinc. "The zinc-deficient girl may not have a regularly established menstrual cycle until age fourteen to seventeen, or the menses may start at thirteen, only to skip for months or even a year," suggests Dr. Carl C. Pfeiffer, the director of the Princeton Brain Bio Center in Skillman, New Jersey. "If placed on vitamin B-6 and zinc [supplements], these patients usually establish a normal menstrual cycle within two to three months."[1]

The Mauve Factor

About 10 percent of normal, nonschizophrenic people (and about 50 percent of schizophrenics) excrete a substance called kryptopyrrole in their urine. This substance, called the "mauve factor," combines biochemically with vitamin B-6 (pyridoxine) and zinc, causing a deficiency of these two nutrients even when dietary intake is normal.

Dr. Pfeiffer claims that a deficiency of zinc and vitamin B-6 is the most common cause of amenorrhea. He and his staff have coined the name "pyroluria" to describe the complex of symptoms that includes pyrroles in the urine. Typically, the patient also has white spots in the fingernails, loss of dreaming or the inability to remember dreams, sweetish breath odor, occasional abdominal pain in the left upper quadrant, constipation, stretch marks on the skin, inability to tan, sensitivity to sunlight, and possible tremors and amnesia. Also, she may have anemia that does not improve with iron but does improve with vitamin B-6.

The dream-recall factor with this condition is so strong that Pfeiffer's staff members know when they have given enough B-6 to the patient: Normal dream recall returns. Although the RDA for B-6 is 2 mg, the Brain Bio staff has found that even "normal" people who don't recall their dreams may need 25 to 50 mg a day if they are to remember dreams, and those with pyroluria who manifest psychopathology may need as much as 2 *grams* a day to keep their urine free of kryptopyrrole, and their minds clear of psychopathological symptoms. According to Pfeiffer, you may have *no* mental illness, but still have this extra need for B-6 and zinc. The zinc, Pfeiffer has found, helps prevent temporary numbness of fingers or toes caused by high doses of B-6.

A Matter of a Pound or Two

It is well known that women who push their bodies to the limit as professional dancers or athletes often have amenorrhea. In 1979, researchers studying women participating in the New York City Marathon found that those weighing the least were the most likely to lack menstrual periods.

Because thinness alone doesn't seem to cut off menstruation, researchers have focused on the *amount* of fat within muscles and under the skin. Women can weigh the same and have very different amounts of body fat. Body fat levels may link the amenorrhea seen in anorexia with that created by overtraining in athletes and dancers. Dr. Richard A. Kunin of San Francisco suggests that body fat must be at least 18 percent of total body composition for normal menstruation to take place. A study of 45 women athletes at Radcliffe College found that 17 percent body fat was the dividing line. The relationship between body fat and the menstrual cycle is so fine-tuned that one or two pounds made the difference between menstruation and amenorrhea for some of these women.[2]

The Diet Connection

In *The Nutrition Detective,* Nan Fuchs describes amenorrhea brought on by imbalanced diets, for example, a diet containing inordinate amounts of vegetables high in carotene (found in carrots, pumpkins, squash, broccoli, and other orange or green vegetables). Eating more protein and reducing the carotene in their diets brought on the women's periods in a short time.[3] Carotene, we must point out, is a very important nutrient for keeping the body cancer-free and strengthening the immune system. But it is possible to overdo anything, even a helpful nutrient.

Another eating indiscretion is a diet too low in fat and protein. The body does need some fat to produce estrogen. Low blood estrogen can lead to amenorrhea.

What's a woman to do? Balance is the key to having healthy menstrual cycles. Eat a variety of grains and vegetables, and a variety of sources of protein, so that even if you are a vegetarian, you eat a combination of foodstuffs that gives you the amino acids, fats, vitamins, and minerals your body needs for all of its life tasks. Our favorite book in this department is the classic *Diet for a Small Planet,* by Frances Moore Lappé (see Selected Bibliography). Another suggestion is to "create a rainbow" at every meal. Is there something green on your plate? Did you eat something orange or yellow today? The color of foods says a lot about its nutrient content. Go for bright foods colored by nature, not laboratory dyes, and you will be on the path to health.

One last caveat in the food department. Whatever you eat must be absorbed by your digestive system in order to bring its nutrient wealth to your body. If you are low in hydrochloric acid, which digests protein in the stomach, proteins will decay when they reach the intestines, leading to gas, bloating, and perhaps constipation, along with malnourishment. If you are low in pancreatic enzymes, your starches will have the same fate. And if your liver doesn't produce enough bile, fats will not be digested adequately. If you are suffering from digestive disturbances along with your amenorrhea, be sure to add digestive enzymes to your supplement regime.

View from the Orient

Nan Fuchs describes the Oriental medical approach to gynecological problems in *The Nutrition Detective.* Fuchs explains to her readers that in the Orient foods are categorized as "hot" and "cold," according to their effect on the body's physiology. Amenorrhea is seen in this Eastern medical system as a blood congestion problem, or a disease of cold nature. Besides acupuncture to stimulate blood circulation, the treatment includes warming herbs and foods. Fuchs, a practicing nutritionist, suggests that her clients eat whole grains, ginger tea, spiced dishes, and miso soup. Miso is soybean paste, and can be stirred into a cup of boiled water one minute before it is to be consumed. Don't boil the miso, itself, or you'll destroy the helpful digestive enzymes it naturally contains.

In Oriental medicine, the liver is in charge of menstruation. The liver produces bile, which is needed to digest fats, and fats are needed to produce estrogen. Also, the liver is responsible for clearing excess estrogens from the body. Western physiology agrees with Eastern philosophy on this point. And we agree with Nan Fuchs that acupuncture is a useful treatment for amenorrhea, or any other menstrual problem.

Thyroid—A Little Too Little

Dr. Broda Barnes, one of the nation's experts on hypothyroidism, describes the importance of the thyroid in regulating menstrual cycles in his book, *Hypothyroidism: The Unsuspected Illness.* He writes, "The thyroid gland is intimately linked with reproduction although all the details of how are still not completely understood. . . . Thyroid secretions in adequate amounts appear to be essential for the development of the egg and for proper ovarian secretions."[4]

One problem with the "thyroid connection" is the difficulty in diagnosing borderline low thyroid function. Laboratory tests can fool the doctor into thinking that the patient is normal. The patient's own testing procedure is often more valuable than any laboratory test for diagnosing a hypothyroid condition. See page 35 for a description of this test.

There are other causes for a low temperature, including starvation, or a deficiency of the pituitary or adrenal gland. According to Dr. Barnes, if thyroid hormone is needed, and you take adequate thyroid treatment, your underarm temperature will rise to normal and your symptoms will disappear. You'll know if you are taking too much thyroid, because your temperature will rise above 98.2°.

Supplements

We've discussed thyroid hormone, B-6 and zinc; vitamin B-12 and folic acid have also been implicated in amenorrhea. Individual B vitamins don't work alone. When you take one, you must also take a B complex so each individual B vitamin can act to its fullest potential. With proper supplementation along with a healthy diet and medical guidance, you can put your inner orchestra into the harmony that nature intended.

IRREGULAR MENSES

In a healthy woman's body, the menstrual flow is approximately the same volume, appears after approximately the same number of days each month, and lasts approximately the same length of time each month. Your menstrual cycle may be wildly different from your best friend's without being abnormal in any way. But if it varies wildly month to month for *you,* if you never know when your period is going to arrive, how long it will last, or how heavy it will be, it's time to see what could be affecting your monthly cycle.

Hovering on the Edge of Hypothyroid

Do you pile on blankets when others are in their shirtsleeves? Is your skin terribly dry, your hair falling out, is your body susceptible to every infection that passes your way? Does it seem to take you forever to do something, and is it difficult to think things through? Are you often confused, depressed, dog-tired or frustrated by poor memory? Maybe your thyroid gland isn't producing as much thyroid hormone as you need.

Malfunction of the thyroid gland, located in the center of your throat, is one frequent cause of menstrual problems. In 1949, Dr. Broda Barnes offered thyroid supplementation to 45 women with irregular menstrual cycles. Thyroid completely regulated the cycles of 41 of the women.[5] You need a doctor's prescription for grains of thyroid extract—it isn't something you pick up over the counter. What is available in health-food stores are the ground-up, dessicated thyroid glands of animals, called protomorphogens or simply glandulars, which are often helpful in such cases. Chiropractors, naturopaths, and other alternative-care practitioners, as well as nutrition-minded physicians, can give you advice regarding your particular case and the possible benefit of glandulars to you.

If your thyroid is hovering on the edge of normal, you can nudge it in the right direction by manipulating your diet, and by taking two convenient products, kelp and the amino acid L-tyrosine.

Iodine is present in minute quantities in your body and is crucial to all your body's various activities, including menstruation. It is stored in the thyroid gland and combines with the amino acid L-tyrosine to form the thyroid hormone thyroxine. Thyroxine regulates the activities of every cell—the speed at which blood absorbs food and the rate at which cells take and convert food to sugar and use the energy from that sugar for all cellular functions. For this process to take place, iodine must be converted to an active form. The body uses protein to manufacture an enzyme, iodine peroxidase, which does the transforming job. Vitamins B-6 and C are also involved in this iodine-tyrosine marriage, as are manganese and choline (a constituent of lecithin).

To create the best possible conditions for your thyroid to function at peak performance and create the quantity of hormone you need for proper menstrual regulation, you need adequate protein daily, supplemented with vitamin B-6, vitamin C, the amino acid L-tyrosine and lecithin or capsules of choline. For an added push, you can take a thyroid glandular.

If You Can't Weight

Another possible cause of irregular menstrual cycles is being overweight. We discuss this in the section on amenorrhea, but we want to also mention it here. We don't know any woman who hasn't been on a diet at one time or another in the recent past, so we assume you may have been, too. Dieting can drastically affect menstruation.

In Munich a few years ago, researchers studied nine normally menstruating young women between the ages of 20 and 29 who were of normal weight, but who dieted for a period of six weeks. The women all lost between 15 and 18 pounds, but the dieting radically affected five of the women's menstrual cycles. Two women stopped menstruating and three stopped ovulating, though their menstruation continued. The researchers concluded that dieting can affect fertility.[6] Apparently it can also cause menstrual irregularities. So, if you're on a strict but temporary diet, wait for the diet to end before exploring why your menstrual periods are no longer like clockwork. They may reappear once you start eating normally again.

In this age of obsessive thinness, it is difficult for women to love the "golden mean," but physiologically that is what our body desires most. The German women in the above study all regained their weight in the six months following the experiment. Remember, though they were "pleased" to have lost weight during the six-week study, they began the experiment at a normal weight. Other studies have shown that when a woman weighs 10 to 15 percent below her normal weight, her periods stop.

If you look in the mirror and say "Ugh!" ask yourself if your reaction is due to an unreasonable image of how you think you should look. If you are unhappy with the way you look because your weight isn't what it is "supposed" to be, you may find benefit in seeing a counselor to work on your self-confidence and self-esteem, rather than continuing to thwart your biology and upset your hormone system with unhappy, unsuccessful diets. You deserve to be healthy! Don't let the power of fashion oppress you.

Life-style Changes

Whether you want to lose weight, gain weight, or simply harmonize your menstrual periods so they are regular and comfortable each month, a wholesome diet is the basis for your self-treatment program. You know the list by now—whole grains (for example, oatmeal for breakfast, 100 percent whole-wheat bread at lunch, and millet, buckwheat groats, or brown rice for dinner), fresh, lightly steamed or raw vegetables, fresh and dried fruits, nuts, seeds, legumes, and tofu (bean curd). If food doesn't contribute to your nutrition, don't spend money on it. See meals as medicine, and medicate yourself with nutritious foods.

Stress reduction is a crucial factor in healing any menstrual problem. Sometimes, the muscles of the back are so constricted owing to stress or trauma that the bones of your spine are moved out of alignment. The changed configuration of muscles and bones may impinge on the nerves leading outward from between the vertebrae. If this occurs to nerves extending into the pelvic organs, the function of your uterus may be affected. In these cases, manipulation by a chiropractor or osteopathic physician may be a beneficial part of your treatment plan for irregular menses.

Simply moving the bones or massaging the contracted muscles isn't enough if your life continues to be so stressful that your muscles tense up again. In fact, no matter what your physical complaint, a case can be made for stress reduction as part of your self-care. Some women find that regular exercise de-stresses them. They attend aerobic dancing classes, run alone or with running clubs, swim, jog, take their dog for a brisk walk, or do any number of activities that force them to breathe deeply and move energetically. Toning pelvic muscles helps your organs work efficiently, and improving blood circulation is a great treatment for any menstrual difficulty.

Other women find that stress reduction is the result of more serene pursuits, such as yoga, meditation, visualization, and listening to music. Many fine tapes are available to help you relax and de-stress. In addition, acupuncture is a known method of relaxation, perhaps because it stimulates the release of endorphins, those self-made opiates that create feelings of calmness and contentment.

TOO PAINFUL MENSES—DYSMENORRHEA

Dysmenorrhea refers to a group of symptoms that have as their common focus severely painful menstruation, and if this is your problem, you don't need anyone to describe it for you. One young woman took to her bed for at least three days a month, bent over in such pain that she couldn't attend classes or go out of the house. If only she had known that relief was possible with a change in her diet, some supplements, and gentle exercises.

Cramps are painful muscle contractions. Even if yours aren't so debilitating that you have to take to your bed, they might stop your mind from thinking in the middle of an examination. As many as 70 percent of American women suffer these monthly pains. Before you embark on a program for natural relief, do get yourself examined by a physician who can rule out diseases and medical conditions such as cancer, endometriosis, pelvic inflammatory disease, and congenital defects of your anatomy that might be causing your pain. You can be especially suspicious of an organic cause if your pain is localized on the right or left side of your pelvis, or if the pain seems to cover the entire abdomen rather than the low, central pelvic area where the uterus is located. If your painful menstruation is a symptom of any of the medical conditions listed above, then your cramps are called secondary dysmenorrhea and will resolve themselves once the underlying organic disorder is corrected.

For about 80 percent of women, however, no organic cause can be found. These cases are called primary dysmenorrhea, and the usual medical treatment is oral contraceptives, other hormones, analgesics, or other drugs. Fortunately, this problem is responsive to natural healing methods, including nutritional supplementation.

Congestion of blood in the uterus has long been recognized as a cause of cramps. Even back in Hippocrates' day, "stagnation of menstrual blood" was considered to be the cause of pain. It was noted that women were frequently relieved of menstrual cramps after delivery of a child, and the logical assumption was that the increase in blood supply to the uterus, which persists after pregnancy, helped to provide enough oxygen and nutrients to the uterine muscles to prevent cramping.[7]

Herbal Remedies

Hippocrates suggested that a woman crouch, bare-bottomed, over steaming combinations of sweet wine, fennel seed and root, and rose oil. If this remedy didn't relieve the pain, it at least must have given her private parts a delicious scent. In the eighteenth century, the ingredients of the steaming brew changed to tansy, hoarhound, wormwood, catnip, and hops. The Latin name for wormwood is Artemisia absinthium. Another member of the Artemisia family, Artemisia vulgaris (mugwort) is used extensively in Chinese healing to this day.

The Chinese treatment is called moxibustion. The herb, called moxa, is bound in slow-burning paper in the shape of open-ended cigars and held near the woman's abdomen to warm the skin and help stimulate blood circulation. While working in an acupuncture clinic in Nanjing, China, Carolyn was taught to use moxibustion in a novel way. A wooden box about the height of a shoe box but shorter and almost square was used. It had a lid, and about three-fourths of the way down inside the box was a wire mesh screen. The doctor broke off several pieces from the moxa stick, lit them, and placed them on the mesh. The woman with cramps rested on a couch, holding the closed moxa box on the skin of her abdomen. The Chinese medical staff believe that the moxa not only warms the pelvic region and improves blood circulation, but that the vapors of that plant have healing properties. The Chinese have experimented with other herbs and have concluded that Artemisia vulgaris has greater healing benefits than others when burned near the skin. If the heat becomes uncomfortable, the box (or the moxa stick, if it is hand-held) is simply lifted farther from the skin surface.

Western herbalists have their own favorite remedies. One is raspberry leaf tea; another is very pointedly called crampbark (Viburnum opulus). Crampbark is taken in combination with other herbs in tea. Laboratory analysis of the herb reveals high doses of vitamin C, which is known to increase capillary permeability, and thereby facilitates the flow of nutrients into muscles and waste products out. We're not sure if that is why crampbark helps menstrual cramps.

If you don't feel like going exotic, you can simply pick up Grandmother's standby, chamomile tea, at any grocery store. Chamomile tea consists of pale, aromatic yellow flowers. If you are allergic to ragweed, skip the chamomile tea, as it can cause an allergic response.

For others, chamomile is a sedative. Chamomile tea contains a good dose of the amino acid tryptophan, which helps you fall asleep effortlessly. For generations it has been taken for intestinal gas, nervousness, insomnia, and cramps.

Make Mine a Mineral

We find mineral deficiencies to be even more significant than vitamin deficiencies as causes of menstrual cramps. Calcium and magnesium are our minerals of choice. Adequate magnesium is necessary for muscles to relax. A lack of magnesium leads to muscle spasm, and to underuse of calcium by the body, even when adequate calcium is consumed. Calcium, in turn, is also needed for proper neuromuscular function. Both calcium and magnesium are considered to be natural tranquilizers, soothing irritated muscles and nerves. Magnesium, in addition, helps the body to use other vitamins, such as C, B complex, and E.

Just as with iron, when magnesium stores are low, the body absorbs more dietary magnesium than when there is plenty already stored away. The phytates in cereal grains and oxalic acid in certain vegetables, such as spinach, can make magnesium unavailable for absorption. Also, cooking and refining of foods can leach out this vital mineral. Or a magnesium deficiency can result from malabsorption owing to liver, pancreas, kidney, or intestinal disease, a high carbohydrate diet, chronic diarrhea, or vomiting.

"I often recommend magnesium for menstrual cramps," Larry Eckstein, M.D., told us. Dr. Eckstein's practice in Santa Monica includes a naturopath-acupuncturist-herbalist, a chiropractor, a nurse practitioner, and other alternative-care specialists. "Sometimes, magnesium has the side effect of causing diarrhea, because it seems to be a bowel irritant. . . . It can be cathartic, but ordinarily it helps to relax the muscles. Magnesium in high doses is in most of the PMS formulas, but I think it's there probably mostly for the menstrual cramping rather than the PMS." Dr. Eckstein recommends that his patients purchase chelated magnesium supplements for better absorption.

Robert J. Peshek is a dentist in Riverside, California. Family health problems that were not solved by conservative, orthodox Western medical care lead Peshek and his family into nutrition, herbs, and other alternative methods of healing. Using his own office laboratory, Peshek has followed the blood chemistries of many patients over the past 16 years and can attest to the benefits of nutritional therapy.

Peshek has found that his patients were relieved of their cramps by the use of magnesium. He claims that four or five chelated magnesium tablets taken when menstrual cramps occur will stop the cramping in 45 minutes, with a lessening of pain felt in 25 minutes. We suspect that having written that, some of you will take 10 tablets, hoping the pain will disappear in half the time! If you happen to be taking antacids rich in magnesium, and magnesium supplements along with other minerals for preventing osteoporosis, and perhaps laxatives such as milk of magnesia, it is theoretically possible to overdose on this mineral. Symptoms include drowsiness, slightly slurred speech, muscle twitching, nausea, flushed skin, heartbeat irregularities, and retention of urine. It gets worse from there, but we assume that with this warning, by the time you feel these symptoms you will be aware that something is wrong and cut back on your magnesium.

Positive Inhibition

Every tissue in the body has within it hormonelike substances called prostaglandins. There are several dozen kinds of prostaglandins, but only a few are biologically active. The ones that affect the smooth muscle and blood flow in the uterus are called PGE-1, PGE-2, PGF-1, and PGF-2. They are potent, powerful, and everywhere: They are formed in every organ from essential fatty acids stored in that organ. Prostaglandins are organ-specific, and when the prostaglandin finishes doing its job, it is quickly destroyed so that it cannot influence the functions of other organs. The need for essential fatty acids (EFA) to re-create or manipulate prostaglandins is a constant necessity in our body.

Sometimes essential fatty acids are called vitamin F because they must come from our diet. The most important essential fatty acid is linoleic acid, which is converted with the help of certain nutrients to prostaglandin E-1. The first step in that conversion is from linoleic acid to gamma linolenic acid (GLA). For children and others having efficient systems, this conversion is a breeze.

For many others, including women who eat high-cholesterol diets, who eat heated or processed oils like margarine, who are under stress, who have diabetes, who drink a good deal of alcohol, or who suffer from an inherited tendency to have allergies resulting in asthma, constant runny nose, or eczema, this prostaglandin conversion is far from easy. In fact, it is downright inefficient. For these folks, less than 1 percent of their dietary linoleic acid may be converted to the GLA form. David Horrobin, an expert on these particular fatty acids, writes that the remaining 99 percent is not wasted, since it can be used for energy, but it doesn't add to the body's needed essential fatty acid stores.

Cis-linoleic acid is found in polyunsaturated vegetable oils like safflower oil, evening primrose oil, linseed oil, borage oil, and black currant oil. These oils are great supplements for the many people whose own bodies have difficulty converting linoleic acid to GLA.

Prostaglandins cause blood vessels to dilate (open), and so reduce blood pressure. Prostaglandins also prevent the development of blood clots, move messages from one brain nerve cell to another,[8] reduce cholesterol, and prevent inflammation. They enhance the health of the skin, the hair, the nails, the liver, the immune system, and the reproductive organs.

But, and this is a big but, all prostaglandins are *not* alike. We've mentioned four different kinds, PGE-1, PGE-2, PGF-1 and PGF-2. PGE-2, PGF-1 and PGF-2 all can *cause* menstrual cramps. They are converted from another fatty acid, arachadonic acid, which is found primarily in animal fat. PGE-1 is the major cramp eliminator. It relaxes smooth muscles, such as those in the uterus walls and around blood vessels. PGE-1 also reduces inflammation. So, the goal of therapy for menstrual cramps is to reduce the manufacture of the three muscle-contracting prostaglandins and increase production of the muscle-relaxing prostaglandin. If your physician has prescribed "prostaglandin inhibitor" type drugs for you in the past, you know that they can be miracle pain relievers. But they inhibit *all* the prostaglandins, even the PGE-1 cramp relievers.

If you want to eliminate your menstrual cramps without drugs, side effects, or visit to the doctor, simply manipulate your dietary intake of substances rich in the raw materials that create PGE-1–type prostaglandins. It's your choice. You can choose cold-pressed polyunsaturated oils for salad dressings, throw out the margarine, lard, red meat, and anything in your cupboard that lists palm oil, coconut oil, or hydrogenated oil of any kind on the label, and, if you can afford it, purchase evening primrose oil, linseed oil, borage oil, or black currant oil for at least three months. In addition, we recommend that you take certain nutrients along with the oils: magnesium, vitamin B-6, zinc, vitamin C, and niacin. These nutrients are used by the body in the all-important set of transformations that change linoleic acid to PGE-1, the cramp reliever.

Decongesting the Abdomen

A diet rich in vegetables and grains, low in saturated fats, and containing the essential supplements mentioned above will relieve your menstrual pains, but let's not stop there. We want to help you become radiantly healthy, not just be pain-free. So we must mention three additional steps you may want to take to envigorate your body, mind, and spirit: exercise, relaxation, and body manipulation.

First, exercise. We include under this category vigorous walking, jogging, and swimming, and also the muscle-stretching, toning effects of yoga. You don't have to pay anyone to teach you this gentle, effective system. There are numerous fine books, even videotapes, that offer adequate instruction.

Exercise generally improves the circulation of blood, reducing congestion in the pelvic region and helping to prevent cramps. Toned, oxygenated muscles work longer before tiring. Choose the exercise that best fits your personal life-style; find something that is convenient and fun so you can commit yourself to doing it at least three times a week, regardless of work pressures, relationship obligations, or weather.

Warm up with stretching, wearing adequate clothing. Swim in warm water. Warm up with room temperature water both before and after you exert yourself. Warm up, inside and out, and your blood vessels will dilate, your blood will flow unimpeded, your muscle fibers will sing as they work, and you will avoid cramps not only in your pelvis, but in your exercising limbs as well.

Relax!

In the medical books that give advice to physicians on pathological conditions, we see footnote references to stress and emotional factors as causes of cramps. Undoubtedly, some women need psychological counseling to cope with their lives, and until they get a handle on their problems, their menstrual cramps will persist. When we are upset, we close up, withdraw, and close in—our shoulders hunch, our fists clench, our jaws tighten. Muscles of our face and our limbs contract, so why not our organs?

Thinking nutritionally, however, stress has other consequences. Stress hampers the turnover from fatty acids to prostaglandins,[9] perhaps because stress impedes our absorption of magnesium and hastens its elimination, and also uses up vitamin C and vitamin B-6 (all of which are needed for converting EFA to PGE-1).

How do you relax when you live the normal American life-style? You *don't* learn to relax by deciding to overhaul your life in one grandiose sweep of the life-style broom. Change, even from bad habits to good ones, is stressful and is best done gradually. Choose one change, like taking the supplements we recommend, every morning and evening. Do it for a week. Do it until it doesn't feel like any more effort than regularly brushing your teeth. Then choose another change, maybe walking for a half hour before starting your work day. Excuses are simply acknowledgments that you don't want to do it. If you were crazy about someone and he invited you to walk with him three mornings a week, somehow you'd get up early and look smashing and go for your walk and still get to work on time.

Notice what you find time to do, and you will discover your true priorities. You may prefer to do a half hour of yoga in the morning to ease yourself into your day, and follow with a videocassette that leads you through a vigorous workout just before dinner. For some, exercise may be the relaxation they need. For others, relaxation is sitting in a hot tub for a half hour, with a candle lit and gentle music in the air. Or putting a comedy on the videocassette deck, snuggling up with a beloved and laughing away the day's cares. Do whatever works for you.

If you would like the help of a professional in learning to relax, we recommend autogenic or biofeedback training. After several sessions with the appropriate professional guide, you will learn to control your own physiology, relaxing blood vessels, muscles, and your nervous system—all without drugs, machines, or anyone else's advice.

Physical manipulation may be useful for you, if any joints in your body are out of alignment. Muscles, ligaments, and nerves cannot function optimally if there is a restriction anywhere in the body. An osteopathic physician who follows the traditions of the profession's founder, Andrew Taylor Still, will be able to release restrictions of muscle and connective tissue. Chiropractors focus mainly on the spine. Menstrual cramps and other menstrual disorders may result where subtle or not-so-subtle contortions of the vertebrae impinge on the nerves that exit the spine to the pelvis. There are subcategories of therapies within both osteopathic and chiropractic methods: Some practitioners do gentle movements, some use vigorous manipulations. Some see the skull and sacrum as one system (the "sacro-occipital technique") and some use machines that send a painless electrical pulse into acupuncture points on the skin to stimulate the body's own healing process.

Ross Trattler, a naturopathic doctor in Hilo, Hawaii, describes the effect of poor body mechanics: "In the woman with normal posture, with strong abdominal muscles and pelvic supports, the female organs are suspended unencumbered within the pelvis. If, however, the abdominal muscles are weakened, or there is an excess lordotic curve in the low back, then the abdominal contents prolapse and put pressure on the pelvic organs. This may result from simple lack of demanding exercises, spinal lesions causing an increase in the lumbar curve, or something as common as the habitual wearing of high-heeled shoes, which increases the lumbar curve. Constipation and "loaded bowel syndrome" may also cause intestinal prolapse. . . . The resultant prolapse interferes with normal blood and lymph flow, resulting in congestion and reduction in local tissue vitality."[10]

You may find relief from your menstrual cramps without resorting to anything besides supplements. Great. In case your body needs a bit more to get you all the way there, we suggest exercise, relaxation, and manipulation.

IUD to Blame?

For 10 horrible months during her 20's, Debbie felt like the fairy-tale mermaid who was given legs so she could marry the prince, except that every step she took was agony. For Debbie, every menstrual period was agony, with pain so severe that she was bent over double, unable to think, move, or work. She gritted her teeth through it, because of the convenience of an intrauterine device (IUD) as a birth control method. Finally, she went back to the clinic that dispensed the device, certain that she had a pelvic infection. There was no infection. The IUD had worked itself out of her uterus and was on its way down the vaginal canal. She chose a diaphragm for her next contraceptive.

Debbie was lucky. An IUD can cause more serious complications than any other contraceptive method, including the Pill. Pelvic inflammatory disease occurs in about 3 percent of IUD users, and it can, if it spreads to the bloodstream, be fatal. Other complications of IUD use include perforation of the uterus (possibly in one in 1,000 users), hemorrhage, and ectopic (tubal) pregnancy. After removal of the device, there is a higher incidence of infertility than for those women who haven't used an IUD. This outcome is thought to relate to the higher incidence of infection: The strings that hang down into the woman's vagina from the end of the device, which allow the woman to check that the IUD is still in place, also provide a convenient pathway for bacteria from the vagina into the uterine cavity.

According to the American Health Foundation, 5 to 15 percent of all IUD users, especially those who have never given birth, return to their doctor to have the IUD removed within the first year, owing to the increased bleeding and cramps that the device causes.

If you have an IUD and suffer from menstrual cramps, why are you punishing yourself? Get a diaphragm or a cervical cap, or keep a full drawer of condoms handy. The spermicide that you use with these barrier methods also helps protect you against sexually transmitted diseases. You have a right to be free of pain, free of disease, and free of guilt when you act responsibly and maturely to protect yourself from an unwanted pregnancy.

TOO MUCH—MENORRHAGIA

You have probably heard of the word "hemorrhage." "Menorrhagia" has a similar meaning. The origin of the word "menorrhagia" is in the Greek words for "month" (*men*) and "to burst forth" (*rhegnynai*). Menorrhagia means unusually long and profuse bleeding during menstruation. Since women don't usually discuss the details of their menstruation with others, there are women who don't realize that their menstrual flow is unusual.

One doctor describes excessive menstrual flow as one in which "double pads must be worn because one soaks through, duration of periods is greater than five days, large clots are passed and more than 12 pads per period are needed."[11] If you fall into this category, don't despair. Like a wound anywhere else in the body, the inner lining of your uterus must be provided with adequate nutrients in order for blood to coagulate, tiny blood vessel walls to contain the flow, and regeneration of tissue to occur. We're going to tell you how, with the proper care, your frantic runs to the bathroom will be over.

Why We Bleed

Ever since viewing those slide shows and films in sixth-grade on female growth and development, you've known that you bleed each month because your uterus prepares a lush, blood-rich cushion for a fertilized egg. When the egg is not fertilized and not implanted in the uterus, various hormones signal the uterus to release the extra blood so the cycle of buildup can begin again. If you are bleeding too profusely each month, some part of the self-regulating mechanism that turns the flow on and off is askew. To better understand how to regulate your monthly flow, you'll need to take a quick look inside and see just what is happening to that overly prolific lining.

The innermost lining of the uterine wall is a mucous membrane called the endometrium. Beneath its surface are tubular glands that can secrete mucouslike substances. Also, some blood vessels reach right up to the border of the lining.

During the first two weeks following menstruation, estrogen from the ovary makes the whole uterine area grow and develop. The glands lengthen, and the blood vessels branch out and increase their presence. A mesh of special fibers appears and interconnects through the area, thickening it. Around Day 14 of the cycle, ovulation occurs.

During the two weeks following ovulation, estrogen diminishes. Sometimes this decrease causes a little bleeding to occur even at this midcycle stage. At the site where the egg bursts through the wall of the ovary a special gland forms, called the corpus luteum. It secretes progesterone, which stimulates the endometrium to more than double its thickness. The tube-shaped glands grow long, swollen and twisty, and secrete a thick mucus. The arterioles (or tiny arteries) in the area coil like long springs, and wear bands of smooth muscle that, when contracted, hold back the blood.

If a fertilized egg implants somewhere on this uterine surface, the corpus luteum will continue to secrete progesterone and the endometrium will continue to develop. If no implantation occurs, then the corpus luteum gets the proper message through hormonal messengers, and deteriorates. As progesterone levels diminish, the endometrium begins to break down and menstrual bleeding begins.

Some coiled arterioles contract, withholding the oxygen-rich blood from the outer border layers of the womb lining. These layers die and slough off. Some of the coiled arterioles break down and release their blood. And some of the tube-shaped glands release their mucous. So, menstrual flow includes blood, endometrial tissue, and mucous secretions.

While some blood vessels are releasing blood, others continue to contract and prevent excessive hemorrhage. The base part of the glands, the arterioles farther from the surface, and the inner layers of the endometrium begin to repair themselves even before menstruation is over.

You can probably visualize easily what nutrients you need to take to control this process: You need something to strengthen the contraction of smooth muscles around the arterioles, to hold back blood; something to heal mucous membranes; something to balance the ebb and flow of estrogen and progesterone. That's it. For some people, the standard medical solution, a D&C or dilatation and curettage, works. Basically, a D&C cleans out the uterine lining by scraping away the outer, discarded layer of the endometrium. Our solution is quite different. But please note that abnormal bleeding, especially after menopause, may be a sign of uterine cancer, so it's best to have a checkup by a gynecologist, regardless of the treatment program you intend to pursue.

Damming the Flow with Thyroid

We have already mentioned in this book the importance of establishing and maintaining thyroid balance, and we will return to this theme repeatedly. Thyroid hormone is in charge of regulating many body processes, including the menstrual cycle, with its reliance on the ebb and flow of estrogen and progesterone.

Dr. Broda O. Barnes has been called Dr. Thyroid because of his pioneering and inspiring research on the functions of the thyroid gland and the hormones it produces. You will be meeting Dr. Barnes, the author of *Hypothyroidism: The Hidden Illness*, throughout this book. Back in 1949, Barnes published a report on his use of thyroid replacement therapy for 50 women suffering excessive menstrual flow. Only two derived no benefit from the treatment. Forty-six resumed periods with normal flow, and two improved somewhat. A study performed at the Mayo Clinic demonstrated that abnormally profuse menstrual flow was a common disturbance among hypothyroid women, and was relieved by using thyroid replacement therapy.

As Dr. Barnes wrote in 1976, "Recently, within a period of a few months, I saw three women who had undergone hysterectomies before the age of twenty-five for excessive bleeding. None had been suspected of having low thyroid function yet each had numerous other symptoms of the disorder—easy fatigability *[sic]*, dry skin, circulatory disturbances—which promptly disappeared with adequate thyroid therapy. The odds are high that needless surgery might have been avoided and these women could have raised families if hypothyroidism had been considered earlier."[12] One problem is that if you are borderline hypothyroid, your menstrual cycle may be affected but doctors may not agree that you need thyroid replacement therapy. According to Barnes, the best test is the temperature test described on page 35.

If you are borderline hypothyroid, you may want to try the animal glandulars mentioned on page 35 before getting a doctor's prescription. If they don't help, you can then go to a doctor and discuss obtaining thyroid.

Also, there are natural substances that can help your body make adequate hormone. Seafood is rich with iodine. So is kelp, a kind of seaweed. Iodine has been used to cure thyroid deficiency since the time of the Incas of South America, the Egyptian pharoahs, and the ancient Chinese. It is an important constituent of the thyroid gland, and is needed to synthesize its hormones. You can buy kelp as tablets or powder. You can use the powder as a seasoning, as you would use salt, or take the tablets with your other supplements.

L-Tyrosine is an amino acid, one of the "building blocks of protein." It is also part of the complex chain of events that form thyroid hormone. Always take amino acids alone, without food or other supplements. You can use a little juice to get them down, but never take amino acids with protein foods, or you're wasting your time and money. Amino acids compete with one another for the biochemical pathways they need to be absorbed and used by the body. The food will fill up the pathways and the amino acid will be simply excreted by your body, unused.

Helping Smooth Muscle Do Its Job

If you are hemorrhaging each month, then the smooth muscle fibers encircling the little uterine arterioles need help contracting. When they contract tightly and properly, they retard the flow of blood. You may wonder how any menstrual blood flows in women in which they work well. The body has its ways! Specifically, the body does not work on an all-or-nothing switch. It selectively allows some arterioles to discharge their contents while others are given the signal to dam it up.

Muscles are composed of protein and essential fatty acids (EFAs). Vitamin E helps form enzymes that are involved in muscle contractions. Potassium, calcium, and magnesium are also involved in maintaining proper muscular contraction. A potassium deficiency can result from a diet of refined foods, "junk foods," and stress—as well as diarrhea, kidney damage, or certain drugs such as diuretics or cortisone.

Since muscle is protein, your diet must contain adequate protein to bring strength to your own muscle cells. If you've been a halfhearted vegetarian, not eating meat but not paying much attention to what you do eat and in what combinations, please purchase *Diet for a Small Planet*, by Frances Moore Lappé (Ballantine, 1982) and combine your nonmeat foods thoughtfully and appropriately. You don't have to eat meat to provide your body with adequate protein, but you do have to eat "the right stuff," and that includes combinations such as rice and beans, and seeds and grains. Since her book was published, Lappé has changed her mind about the importance of consuming these combinations at the same meal. However, a healthy diet includes these nutrient-rich foods frequently.

In the section on dysmenorrhea (page 80) we go into great detail about substances called prostaglandins. They are similar to hormones and are produced liberally throughout the body to regulate many biochemical functions. They can help conception, induce labor, cause abortion, reduce blood pressure, remove blood clots, and cause smooth muscles to contract. Prostaglandins are part of the brain, and are also thought to move messages from nerve to nerve. The function we are interested in here is their control of smooth muscle contraction. Muscles, as we mentioned, are composed of essential fatty acids (EFA) among other things. EFAs, especially the EFA called linoleic acid, is transformed in the body to make certain prostaglandins. So you need EFAs for both muscle form and muscle function.

The best sources of EFAs are polyunsaturated vegetable oils, such as safflower oil, evening primrose oil, linseed oil, borage oil, and black currant oil. Whatever oil you choose, be sure it is cold-pressed. Do not heat or cook with it. Swallow it straight from the refrigerator, either masked in tomato or other juice, or in a salad dressing of your own concoction. Heating EFAs destroys their potency as prostaglandin synthesizers.

Part of the pathway from linoleic acid to prostaglandins includes the vitamin B complex, particularly B-6. Magnesium and vitamin C are also a part of this conversion process. In the sections on PMS and menstrual cramps (dysmenorrhea) we emphasize the importance of PGE-1, the prostaglandin that relaxes smooth muscle. You don't need more of that in the case of menorrhagia. But PGE-1 is a stage in the synthesis of other prostaglandins, and these later forms (PGE-2, PGF-1, and PGF-2) all contract smooth muscle. Nutrition-minded health practitioners have found that EFAs can help with all menstrual difficulties, from too little bleeding to too much. See what these supplements do for you. They won't hurt you. The worst that can happen is that they do nothing.

Healing and Repair

Between buildup and break-down of the uterus comes the stage of repair. There is no question but that vitamin A is the premier nutrient when it comes to healing and repairing mucous membranes. Dominick Bosco describes vitamin A's role as follows: "In order for a wound to heal, new collagen must be formed and linked to hold new tissue together. That linking is dependent upon vitamin A." Women with menorrhagia from no other apparent cause have been found to have low vitamin A levels in their blood. Bosco reports one study in which 52 women with abnormal bleeding were given 30,000 I.U. of vitamin A twice a day for 35 days. The fate of 12 was unknown. For 23, the menstrual flow returned to normal, and 14 others saw improvement in their condition.[13]

Vitamin A is great for mucous membranes, but it isn't the only vitamin useful for healing the endometrium. Bioflavonoids, found in the white pulpy portion of citrus fruits and the dark outer leaves of plants, also have potent healing powers: They strengthen the tiny capillaries that form the bridges between our arteries and our veins. They were discovered thanks to the bleeding gums of a friend of Dr. Albert Szent-Gyorgyi, who won the 1937 Nobel Prize for his discovery of vitamin C. In 1936, while he was still busy isolating pure ascorbic acid, he thoughtfully provided his friend with some of an early preparation of the substance. Szent-Gyorgyi knew that this preparation helped stop bleeding. As expected, the bleeding stopped. By the time the friend's bleeding problem recurred, Szent-Gyorgyi had purified the vitamin—but the purified form didn't work. What did work was an "impurity" in the earlier extract, the bioflavonoids, which the scientist recognized, extracted, and then gave to his friend again.

In his enthusiasm, Szent-Gyorgyi named the "impurity" vitamin P, but later it was shown not to be a true vitamin. Other researchers, however, have found bioflavonoids to be effective in a number of healing ways, particularly in cases of capillary fragility. Capillaries are minute blood vessels, one cell wide. Veins move used blood from the capillaries to the heart, and arteries move freshly oxygenated blood from the heart to the capillaries. It is in the capillaries that life-giving, life-preserving nutrients are passed from the bloodstream to the body's cells, and the waste products of cell metabolism are passed from the cells back into the bloodstream. When capillaries are fragile, instead of nutrients and waste flowing in and out, the blood, itself, bursts through. A bruise forms. Women who are easy bruisers need to strengthen their capillary walls.

Although bioflavonoids are usually associated with citrus fruits such as lemons, grapefruits, and oranges, they are also found in buckwheat and other grains. It is rare to find someone with a clear-cut bioflavonoid deficiency, but more subtle symptoms—such as easy bruising and bleeding gums—are signs that the woman might need more bioflavonoids than she is getting in her diet.

There also seems to be some evidence that bioflavonoids can alter hormone synthesis. In 1974, scientists working at the University of California at Irvine reported in *Science* magazine that they had found some bioflavonoids that inhibited the synthesis of estrogens in humans. Besides their role as controllers of capillary wall strength, bioflavonoids seem to be able to influence hormone production.

Six years earlier, however, the FDA had forced all bioflavonoids produced by pharmaceutical companies to be withdrawn from the market, claiming that a review of the literature on the subject undertaken by a panel of the National Academy of Sciences/National Research Council had convinced the agency that the substance was ineffective "for any condition." Doctors could no longer prescribe the substance, but health-food stores could continue to sell it over the counter. Confused? Such is the world of political power, nutrition, and science, and American agencies mandated to bridge the three arenas. We side with the physicians and researchers whose many patients benefited from using bioflavonoids between 1936 and 1968. We suggest that you use bioflavonoids yourself and make up your own mind. As you observe the effects of bioflavonoids and other supplements on your menstrual cycles, be aware that your body is being nudged, not kicked, in the direction of health. It may take two or three cycles or more for you to see substantial improvement. Give nature a chance to do it her way, at her speed.

There are many different flavonoids, at least 61 in citrus fruits alone. Not all of these are biologically active in humans. Those that are active are called bioflavonoids; the more common ones are rutin and hesperidin. Less commonly known flavonoids such as quercetin, myricetin and kaempferol have been shown to help prevent cataracts and protect foods from oxidation. Certain others, including nobiletin and tangeretin, can stimulate enzymes that detoxify our body from drugs and carcinogenic chemicals.

According to bioflavonoid researcher Dr. R. C. Robbins, certain bioflavonoids from citrus fruits are even stronger antiinflammatory agents than cortisone, and others prevent the clumping of red blood cells. Although this sounds like the opposite of what you, who are suffering from excessive bleeding, would want to take into your body, in fact, Swedish researchers found that excess aggregation of red blood cells actually slows wound healing.[14]

Think Zinc for Healing

No discussion of healing nutrients would be complete without mentioning zinc. Zinc is involved in cell division and in the growth and repair of injured tissue. Zinc seems to accumulate in tissues where healing is taking place. When zinc is deficient, wounds heal slowly.

During the past decade, research has revealed an interesting interaction between zinc and vitamin A: When zinc is deficient, and then given as a supplement, vitamin A metabolism improves. That's why both these two wound-healing agents are on the essential supplement list for excess menstrual bleeding.

A more pronounced zinc deficiency causes dermatitis (skin inflammation), retarded growth, retarded sexual development, impaired sexual function, poor night vision, impaired immunity, and susceptibility to infections, as well as poor wound healing. Mental disturbance and loss of hair have also been reported in people with a severe zinc deficiency.

Although we sometimes recommend taking minerals with meals to avoid gastrointestinal discomfort, studies show that zinc is best absorbed if taken on an empty stomach. A feeling of nausea is, however, a common side effect of zinc, but taking zinc with a carbonated beverage may help relieve stomach discomfort. If you experience nausea, try a little zinc with a little soda water—but not soda pop.

If you're one who just *has* to take it with meals or you'll never remember to take it at all, fine—impaired absorption is preferable to no absorption. Take that zinc with meat or fish, not with a meal of whole grains of any sort. The worst offenders inhibiting zinc absorption are fiber and phytates, both found in grains and beans.

As you figure out your supplement schedule, keep one other important bit of information in mind: don't take zinc at the same time as calcium or iron. These two minerals interfere with zinc absorption.

Now the question is, what form of zinc should you buy? There is a controversy among zinc researchers regarding the best form of zinc to take. Zinc doesn't just pop through your intestinal wall by itself. It needs a helper, a carrier molecule called a ligand, to traverse the cellular barrier between the inside of the intestine and the bloodstream. Some researchers swear that the best ligand is citrate, and others put their money on picolinate. We have had good results with each type, but the picolinate form is more expensive.

A surprisingly large number of Americans are deficient in zinc. Teenage girls, middle-class children, and the elderly in various sites around the country have been surveyed and found lacking in zinc. Obviously, poor choice of foods, or poverty and subsequent inability to afford meat and fish, two good sources of zinc, are common causes. Crohn's disease, which causes malabsorption in the small intestine; kidney disease; and trauma resulting from burns, surgery, psoriasis, and even stress have also been demonstrated to cause zinc deficiency.

Iron to Replace What's Lost

Back in the days when supplements were a dirty word to any self-respecting medical professional, iron was accorded the special status as an "essential supplement for women." It has been estimated that the mean menstrual loss of iron for women is about 0.6 to 0.7 mg per day. We go into greater detail about iron in Chapter 8, on pregnancy. Please refer to that discussion. An iron supplement is a good idea if you are suffering from excessive menstrual bleeding; take it with vitamin C but not with vitamin E.

If you want to add dietary sources of iron, which of course is a very good idea, eat more dried fruits, especially peaches and raisins, eggs, green leafy vegetables, fish, poultry, liver (if you can obtain meat that is raised without drugs and fed fodder without pesticides and herbicides) and blackstrap molasses. A tablespoon of molasses in boiling water makes a tasty hot drink in the morning. Or add the molasses to hot cereal. It's true that the cereal contains phytates, which bind the iron. Our view is, some is better than none. Look for a variety of sources instead of relying on just one or two.

Mirror, Mirror on the Wall, Am I Low in B Complex?

Look at your mouth and tongue in the mirror. Do you have cracks around the corners of your mouth? Is your tongue thick and red? These signs plus excessive menstrual bleeding might well indicate a need for more vitamin B complex. The late Carlton Fredericks, working backward from symptom to cause, pointed out that excessive bleeding can be the result of a hormone imbalance.[15] Imbalance doesn't always simply mean that too much or too little is produced. The body may be producing the appropriate quantity of estrogen, but the liver may not be able to regulate how much of the usable form is available to the body. The liver needs B complex vitamins to metabolize the elemental estrogen produced by the ovary, so that the body's cells can respond to the hormone.

One of the best dietary sources of B complex is brewer's yeast, which you can sprinkle on popcorn, stir into tomato juice, add to breakfast cereal (especially hot cereal after it is cooked), or buy as tablets.

If you are going to go to the trouble and expense of purchasing and using B complex vitamin supplements, we suggest that you eliminate sugar from your diet completely. When your body is working in vibrant good health, some sugar isn't going to do you serious harm. Now, however, when you are doing all you can to stop your excess bleeding and get your body back into balance, eating sugar is as silly as hitting yourself on the head. Sugar steals B vitamins from your system and gives nothing in return.

Other Supplements

Choline and inositol are members of the B complex that may or may not be vitamins in their own right. Although enough research hasn't been done to prove that designation, there is enough research to prove their usefulness. They are called the lipotrophic factors, and as the "lipo-" prefix suggests, they are involved in fat metabolism. Estrogen is a fat-soluble hormone. Choline and inositol help the liver metabolize the hormone.

Choline may improve your memory, too, which is a nice bonus if that has been a problem for you. Choline is a precursor of acetylcholine, which transmits nerve impulses from one nerve to another in the brain. B vitamins plus choline help the transmission of impulses from nerves to muscles and also affect muscle strength. So choline has a second important role in countering menorrhagia: It helps the muscles around the blood vessels in your uterus become strong enough to retard the flow of blood each month.

Vitamin C is another supplement we recommend for menorrhagia, because of its role in keeping the liver healthy. It is also well documented that vitamin C strengthens capillary walls, and is intimately involved in the health of your body's collagen, a protein that forms the fibrous connective tissue that basically holds the body together. As we strengthen the uterine lining and help it to repair and rebuild itself during each menstrual cycle, we certainly want healthy, strong collagen and capillaries. Vitamin C, along with bioflavonoids and vitamin A, is an important supplement for that double job.

Vitamin K (think "*k*oagulation") is the prime vitamin for coagulating blood and stopping hemorrhage. It is not sold over the counter, but it is available in certain foods, such as cabbage, seaweeds, alfalfa, green and leafy vegetables, egg yolks, safflower oil, and blackstrap molasses.

The last supplement that we recommend for menorrhagia is vitamin E. It is used by the body to form the core of muscle cells and to build enzymes that are needed for muscle contraction. Vitamin E is also essential for proper functioning of the liver, which needs vitamin E to produce certain enzymes which it uses to metabolize hormones.

Self-Treatment

Naturopathic doctor Ross Trattler of Hilo, Hawaii, suggests that women suffering from menorrhagia apply ice packs to their pubic region or lower back. Ice, of course, causes blood vessels to contract. You can also apply hot compresses at the same time to your legs and feet. This facilitates removal of blood from the pelvic region to the extremities. But, this approach requires stoic dedication. Try vitamins, first.

PREMENSTRUAL TENSION SYNDROME (PMS)

> She has two different sorts of mood. One day she is all smiles and happiness . . . another day, there'll be no living with her.
> —Simonides, *An Essay on Women*
> sixth century B.C.

What To Do

There are a number of supplements, besides those already mentioned, that are useful for eliminating PMS. Some supplements are needed because of biochemical interactions among nutrients, such as those among vitamin D, magnesium, calcium, zinc, manganese, and vitamin C. Other nutrients can help clear up specific PMS complaints, such as the forgetfulness of PMS type D, which may be countered by choline. Choline is considered a "brain food," because of its proven ability to improve learning retention, but its main role is as a fat emulsifier, and it does a great job of clearing fatty deposits from the liver. We make a strong case for improving liver function in the overall treatment of menstrual problems, and choline is an integral part of any PMS-oriented treatment program.

Antioxidants like vitamins A and E and the mineral selenium may prevent damage by the harmful biochemical process known as oxidation. Vitamins A and E also have roles in PMS prevention, related to their interactions in the multiple biochemical conversions that lead to prostaglandin synthesis.

First of All, Record Yourself

If you feel plagued by monthly depression that seems unreasonable as well as unbearable, do not despair! Buy yourself a day-at-a-glance log book, take a pencil in hand, and begin the most important diary of your life. Each day, write down everything you eat and drink. And we mean everything. That includes the peanuts from the candy machine between classes, the cup of coffee on your 10 o'clock break, the bag of popcorn while watching the late-night movie—everything.

With a red pencil, mark down any PMS symptoms you experience during the two weeks prior to your period's arrival and the time they bother you, for example, "Burst into tears at 3:00 P.M. at the sight of a scrawny cat in a garbage can." And so on.

With a blue pencil note the time you took to exercise, and the kind of exercise: "Walked one half hour," "Jogged 20 minutes."

Don't use this journal for recording any other activities or thoughts, so you'll have plenty of room to record your eating, exercise, and mood patterns. Over the next couple of months, your diary will make illuminating reading. The diary pages tell you where you're at, now, and indicate where you need to go. For your convenience, we list some of the most common symptoms of the different types of PMS in the Daily Supplement Dose Advisory at the end of the chapter.

This book is about the nutritional underpinnings for emotional and physical well-being. The best treatment of PMS works on three fronts: improving nutrition, reducing stress, and taking adequate exercise. This is a book about supplements, so we will just mention in passing the need for regular exercise and stress reduction.

Swimming in warm water is a lovely, body-lulling way to be caressed by your environment on days when you don't want anything human within arm's reach; it can help reduce the tension and congestion of premenstrual days. If you want your exercise to do double duty as a bone builder during your premenopausal years, you'll need some fast, hard, feet-on-the-pavement walking, jogging, or dancing as well.

Carolyn, who used to hate exercise as a "waste of time," now is addicted to a half-hour walk in her neighborhood before delivering her toddler to childcare. Carrying Natanya in a backpack since she was seven months old has served the same purpose as carrying weights. Now Carolyn's back is stronger and her daughter is the pleased recipient of a daily walk with her mother.

Stress reduction techniques abound; if you're the private type, you can buy a good book, or an audiotape to use in the car or at home. There are videocassettes that help you retrain your mind to let go of your cares and relax your way to health. And you can choose from myriad specialists to massage you, counsel you, Rolf you, Hellerwork you, Trager you, analyze you, and teach you to stretch your way to well-being.

Dr. Susan Lark, who cured her own PMS and, in the process, gathered enough great ideas to fill one of the very best books on the subject that we've found (see Selected Bibliography) has a suggestion for women who are too busy to meditate for 20 minutes to half an hour: Simply focus your eyes on the second hand of your watch for 15 seconds of total concentration. Notice how much slower and calmer your breathing becomes.

"As we have strayed farther from nature," writes Dr. Guy Abraham, "our health has paid the price." A return to a balanced life-style of healing nutrients, exercise, and relaxation is the most easily obtainable treatment for premenstrual syndrome. Best of all, it's within your own power to treat yourself.

Don't reproach yourself if you aren't willing or able to revolutionize your life overnight. Commit yourself to a goal of three hours a week of exercise, not an unreasonable target. Take a short walk every day. Good health means good attitude, and a good attitude is one of self-acceptance. Choose those changes that you are willing to make, and leave the rest for the future, when conditions, finances, and your own inclinations allow you to do more for your well-being.

Eat to Heal

Some natural foods have a downside for some people. If these foods don't bother you, there's no reason to limit your intake. Potato skins, tomatoes, green peppers, and eggplant contain solanine, a substance that causes some people's arthritis to flare up. Spinach, rhubarb, cranberries, chard, and beet leaves contain oxalic acid, which is great for treating hemorrhage, since it reduces the blood's coagulation time, but also has an unfortunate ability to make calcium unavailable to the body. If you love any of the above vegetables, be sure to accompany the meal with extra calcium sources such as another dark-green, leafy vegetable, yogurt, sardines, or dried peas or beans. Why the food list on page 95? White sugar and white flour add calories but don't offer nutrition in the balance. In white enriched flour, a few of the many essential nutrients in the grain are replaced, but the amounts are not comparable to what has been removed. White sugar depletes the body's B vitamins, as well as leading to the "sugar crazies." When sugar cravings hit, munch rice crackers with just-the-fruit, no-sugar-added jam, or Kashi, a seven-grain puffed breakfast cereal, or eat some vanilla Rice Dream, which tastes like vanilla ice cream but is made with rice and without refined sweeteners.

The Healthy Woman's Diet

AVOID ENTIRELY

White sugar
White flour
Lard, partially hydrogenated vegetable shortening, visible fat on
meat
Caffeine
Salt

AS LITTLE AS POSSIBLE

Milk, ice cream, cheese, butter
Alcohol
Red meat

DAILY RAINBOW

Whole grains—yellow millet and corn, brown rice, wheat and rye
Legumes—green peas, beans, and lentils
Green and leafy vegetables—broccoli, kale, collard greens, mustard
greens, chard
Orange fruits and vegetables—carrots, squash, cantaloupe, sweet potato
Red fruits and vegetables—apples, cabbage, tomatoes, strawberries

OIL

Safflower oil—eat a couple of tablespoons each day, on a salad or added
to apple or grape juice to hide the taste. Don't cook it.

Salt should not be on the shopping list of someone who is bloated. If you crave salt, use naturally fermented soy sauce, called tamari, for seasoning food and cooking. A quarter teaspoon of tamari has the seasoning power of one teaspoon of salt, yet contains only 270 mg of sodium compared to 2,000 mg in salt. Or make yourself a cup of miso soup. Boil some water, pour the water in a cup, add a teaspoon of miso, and stir until the miso dissolves into a nourishing liquid refreshment that will satisfy your salt craving. Don't boil the miso itself, for this will destroy the good digestive enzymes it contains.

Some nutritionists warn that too much protein pulls minerals away from the body. Meat may also contain traces of steroids, antibiotics, and other drugs injected into the animal during its lifetime. Furthermore, the saturated fats in meat stimulate the growth of certain intestinal bacteria that take inactive forms of estrogen and convert them to active forms, contributing to all the symptoms associated with PMS type A, such as anxiety, irritability, and moodiness.

Dairy products have 10 times more calcium than magnesium, which causes biological havoc in several ways. Bear in mind that the more calcium you eat, the more magnesium you need. The more magnesium you eat, the less calcium you need. High calcium levels make it more difficult for the body to assimilate magnesium, so you need more just to stay in the normal range. Magnesium, however, *helps* calcium absorption and the placement of calcium into the bones, where it belongs.

Dr. Penny Wise Budoff was one of the first physicians to write a book for the lay public on the subject of menstrual difficulties. In *No More Menstrual Cramps and Other Good News* (see Selected Bibliography), Budoff noted that eliminating caffeine led to marked reduction in PMS symptoms for her patients. In 1985, Annette MacKay Rossignol published a study showing that women who drank 4½ to 15 cups of caffeine-containing beverages a day had a greater likelihood of severe PMS symptoms than women who drank fewer caffeinated beverages.

If you need a morning pick-me-up, Dr. Susan Lark suggests the following drink: Boil two teaspoons of grated licorice root together with two teaspoons of grated ginger in a quart of water for five minutes, then let the brew steep for 15 minutes. Drink only one cup per day, she advises, and store the rest in the refrigerator. If all you want is a warm, dark beverage, use Cafix, Postum, or Pero, or some other powdered, grain-based instant drink. Also, check out herbal tea packages for a "No Caffeine" statement; regular dark teas may contain as much as or more caffeine than coffee.

Alcohol, like sugar, depletes your body of B vitamins. Alcohol is also toxic to the liver, and may deplete the body of magnesium, another PMS fighter. Choose mineral water on the rocks with a twist of lemon or lime at parties. When you're facing social pressures to eat or drink unhealthy substances, remember that those who are pressuring you won't have to live with the consequences.

The grains we recommend in The Healthy Woman's Diet contain high quantities of B complex and E vitamins, and the dark, leafy vegetables contain good quantities of minerals like magnesium, zinc, iron, and chromium. Fruits and vegetables also provide the vitamin C and A needed to fuel the important transformation of linoleic oil to prostaglandin E-1. Safflower oil is a convenient source of linoleic acid. Don't cook it or eat it together with hardened fats and heated oil.

Supplements

A number of physicians have developed and market their own supplement formulas for coping with PMS. Dr. Guy Abraham's Optivite® contains digestive enzymes in addition to large doses of vitamins and minerals. Dr. Sandra Cabot has created PMT-eze, which contains European and Native American herbs as well as vitamins and minerals. Dr. Susan Lark's formula lacks digestive aids, but otherwise contains the same vitamins and minerals, in lower doses, as Dr. Abraham's. Her supplements can be ordered by mail (see For Further Information). In fact, most supplement manufacturer's have jumped onto the bandwagon of providing women with a formula especially for PMS.

If you want to purchase the supplements individually, we have listed the dosages we recommend in The Daily Supplement Dose Advisory below. You may, however, be able to save money by buying the prepared formulas. Compare the cost of prepared formulas versus individual supplements at your local health-food store. Buying a high-quality formula especially created to treat PMS is generally a better investment.

Daily Supplement Dose Advisory

ABSENT MENSTRUATION

Vitamin B-6—up to 100 mg
B complex—up to 50 mg
Zinc—up to 50 mg elemental zinc
Thyroid hormone—dosage varies according to body temperature; Must be prescribed by physician

IRREGULAR MENSES

Vitamin B complex—up to 100 mg
Vitamin B-6—up to 100 mg
Vitamin C—up to 5 grams
Zinc—up to 50 mg elemental zinc
Lecithin—one tablespoon or equivalent capsules
Thyroid glandular—as directed on label
Kelp—one tablet with meals

PAINFUL MENSTRUATION

Magnesium—up to 800 mg
Calcium—up to 1,000 mg
Vitamin E—up to 1,000 I.U.
Essential fatty acids—safflower oil (several teaspoons), or evening primrose oil (1,250 mg up to 3 times a day) or borage oil (6 capsules per day) or linseed oil (1,250 mg up to 3 times a day), or black currant oil (as directed on label).
Vitamin B complex—up to 100 mg
Vitamin B-6—up to 100 mg
Zinc—up to 50 mg elemental zinc

TOO MUCH—MENORRHAGIA

Thyroid hormone—advice of physician
Kelp—several tablets daily

L-tyrosine—up to 1 gm
Iron—up to 115 mg daily, in a tablet combined with other compounds
  such as vitamin C, zinc, copper, or magnesium
Zinc—up to 50 mg elemental zinc
Calcium/magnesium—up to 1,000 mg calcium; 800 mg magnesium
Vitamin A—up to 25,000 I.U.
Bioflavonoids—up to 2 gms
Vitamin C—up to 5 gms
Vitamin E—up to 800 IU
Vitamin B complex—up to 100 mg
Vitamin B-6—up to 200 mg extra
Essential Fatty Acids—see dosages under Painful Menstruation, above
Lipotrophics (choline/inositol)—up to 500 mg

PMS

If you fall into two categories, do not duplicate doses of any nutrient.
Start this supplement regimen as soon as you begin menstruating and
carry it out through a complete cycle before attempting higher dosages.

Anxiety
Vitamin B complex—50–100 mg of major B vitamins
Vitamin B-6—100 mg
Magnesium—800 mg

Bloating
Magnesium—800 mg
Iron—up to 115 mg
Vitamin A—10,000 I.U.
Zinc (elemental)—50 mg
Vitamin E—800 I.U.

Cravings
Magnesium—800 mg
Essecntial fatty acid—see dosages under Painful Menstruation, above.
Chromium—200 mg.

Depression
Vitamin B-6—100–200 mg
Iron—up to 115 mg
Vitamin A—10,000 I.U.
Vitamin E—800 I.U.
L-tyrosine (morning)—500 mg
L-tryptophan (bedtime)—500–3,000 mg.
Lipotropic Factors (choline and inositol)—as directed on bottle.

FOR ALL CATEGORIES OF PMS

Beta carotene—up to 150 mg

Vitamin B complex—50 mg of major B vitamins

Vitamin C—at least 5,000 mg or to bowel tolerance

Calcium—1,200 mg

Iodine (available as SSKI [potassium iodide] from Upsher-Smith Laboratories, Minneapolis)—300 mg or 1 dropperful SSKI in ½ glass of liquid.

Multimineral containing at least zinc, copper, manganese, potassium, and selenium

Chapter Six:

Contraception

Due to—Presence of externally administered estrogen, to a lesser extent progesterone.
Solution—Switch contraceptive method, take supplements.
Supplements—Folic acid; vitamin B complex, vitamin B-6, vitamin C, vitamin E, zinc, multiminerals.

This chapter is about the supplements that you need if you use an intrauterine device (IUD) or birth control pills. But first we want to say something about the safer and healthier methods of contraception. Barrier methods of birth control such as the condom, cervical cap, or diaphragm used with spermicide offer excellent protection without any of the serious potential dangers of the IUD and the Pill. In fact, these methods offer you important benefits, such as some measure of protection against infectious diseases. If you feel uncomfortable with the idea of having to put in a birth control device soon before intercourse, you may derive benefit from the writings of Dr. Gerald Jampolsky, (*Love Is Letting Go of Fear,* Bantam, 1981), Nathaniel Branden (*If You Could Hear What I Cannot Say: Learning to Communicate with the Ones You Love,* Bantam, 1983) and Dr. David Viscott (*The Viscott Method: A Revolutionary Method for Self-Analysis and Self-Understanding,* Pocket Books, 1985). Or you may wish to investigate one of the forms of natural birth control.

THE IUD (INTRAUTERINE DEVICE)

The IUD is the contraception method fraught with the greatest health dangers for women. Some of the complications associated with use of an IUD can be fatal, such as pelvic inflammatory disease (PID), or perforation of the uterus. We cannot recommend this form of birth control to anyone. Please read our discussion of the IUD in the section "Painful Menstruation" in Chapter 5.

THE PILL

Birth control pills (BCPs) are popular the world over as an effective and convenient way of preventing pregnancy. It is estimated that about 55 million women, including as many as 10 million in the United States, use the Pill. BCPs work by tricking the body's hormone system into thinking the body is already pregnant. The brain doesn't send a monthly message to the ovaries to stimulate the development of eggs, so ovulation does not usually take place. Since the hormones have also made the uterine wall inhospitable to a fertilized egg, if ovulation and fertilization should by chance occur, the egg cannot implant and pregnancy will still be thwarted. In addition, BCPs make a woman's cervical mucus become thick, which serves as a barrier to the entrance of sperm.[1]

Most women use a combination pill that includes both estrogen and progestin, a form of progesterone. A "minipill" is also available, which contains only progestin. This pill does not prevent ovulation, but does prevent the fertilized egg from implanting in the uterine wall. The minipill also creates a cervical mucus "plug" that blocks out sperm.

The list of potential health effects of the Pill is rather striking. Obviously, with so many women regularly using this method, the statistical risk of any one woman's suffering an adverse effect is relatively small. If you are young and in good health, you may have no side effects whatsoever and wonder what all the fuss is about. Some women, however, have died as a direct result of using birth control pills, owing to the Pill's effects on the cardiovascular system. It makes sense to inform yourself of the numerous potential physiological effects of the Pill on specific organs and on your nutritional needs.

In general, the longer women use the Pill, the greater the chance that serious health effects could result. For example, the risk of developing a noncancerous liver tumor is one in one million if the Pill is used for less than one year, but after five years of Pill use, the risk increases to one in 2,000.

Nutritional Effects of the Pill

If a drug did not affect our biochemistry, scientists would call it a placebo and we would call it a gyp. In the case of birth control drugs, we might also call ourselves pregnant! The birth control pill, because it toys with the body's delicately balanced hormone system, very definitely affects our biochemistry, and the longer we take it, the greater is the overall tinkering that occurs. Let's look, one by one, at the vitamin and mineral changes known to occur to Pill users, and then we'll offer our recommendations for supplementation.

Vitamin A

Levels of vitamin A rise in the bloodstream and fall in the liver of women taking estrogen-containing oral contraceptives. In one study of Pill users, vitamin A levels in the blood were measured as high as 80 percent above the amount found in those not using the Pill. Some observers believe that this increase means that A supplementation is unnecessary, while others believe that a redistribution of vitamin A out of the liver and into the blood signifies a greater, rather than a lesser, need for the nutrient.[2] There is some evidence that birth control pills seem to enhance the body's ability to transform dietary carotene into vitamin A; since carotene is readily available in foods such as sweet potatoes, cantaloupe, winter squash, and carrots, as well as the less popular dark-green and leafy vegetables, we feel that a vitamin A supplement isn't necessary, as long as care is taken to support the liver function by including an orange-colored fruit or vegetable in your daily diet.

Vitamin B-6

Women on the Pill may report feeling depressed, melancholy, nauseated, or bloated. Some women complain of painful, tingling hands and others notice a loss of sex drive. These side effects probably are due to a depletion of vitamin B-6 (pyridoxine). As many as 20 percent of oral contraceptive users have clear biochemical signs of B-6 deficiency, and many others may have an increased need for this vitamin that isn't detectable in ordinary laboratory tests. It is suspected that estrogen in the Pill causes either an increased need for vitamin B-6, or a decreased ability to absorb it.

B-6 plays numerous roles in body chemistry. It is vital for energy production, fat and protein metabolism, mineral absorption, brain function, and red blood cell production. B-6 is essential for the conversion of the amino acid methionine to taurine, which acts in your brain to decrease tension and elevate your mood, and is also involved in the metabolism of the amino acid tryptophan, which is converted to serotonin, a brain neurotransmitter that has been called "the calming chemical."[3] The extra estrogen provided by the Pill lowers B-6 levels, leading to an interference with tryptophan and taurine metabolism. Deficiency of B-6 can prevent your body from creating enough of the biochemicals that give you a happy feeling, leading to depression, irritability, and extreme sensitivity to pain.

As has often been pointed out, however, "Not *all* women become depressed when using oral contraceptives. And of those who do, not *all* depression is necessarily due to pyridoxine deficiency. But among women on the Pill who also have a pyridoxine deficiency, the administration of pyridoxine supplements usually alleviates the depression."[4] The same holds for all the other symptoms noted above. They may not be due to B-6 deficiency, but if they are, B-6 supplementation will noticeably improve them.

B-6 also is an essential factor in carbohydrate metabolism, which is why a Pill-created B-6 deficiency can cause too much glucose (blood sugar) in the blood. This condition has been called "chemical diabetes." In one study, vitamin B-6 supplements of 25 mg a day allowed women to metabolize glucose efficiently and relieved other symptoms of metabolism imbalance, including depression, anxiety, and loss of sexual appetite.[5] Similar results have been achieved with both larger and smaller doses.

It's apparent that the RDA for B-6, which is only 2 mg, is far too low for a woman on birth control pills. Although some unsubstantiated reports of peripheral neuropathy (such as tingling in the fingers and toes) have been reported in people taking enormous doses of B-6 for extended periods of time, there is little risk to a Pill user taking a B-6 supplement of 25 to 100 mg a day, and there is the potential for much benefit, *especially* if she is feeling depressed or bloated.

In addition, make sure your diet includes plenty of *whole* grains (brown rice rather than white rice, and 100 percent *whole*-wheat bread rather than breads that are sold as "wheat bread" but actually contain a large proportion of white flour; they are natural sources of all the B vitamins. You may want to take brewer's yeast in powder form or capsules as well, but not if you suspect you suffer from a yeast infection.

The Other B Vitamins

Some studies of Pill users show no signs of deficiency of the other B vitamins, while others have documented significant abnormalities in thiamin (B-1), riboflavin (B-2), cobalamin (B-12), and, especially, folic acid.

Both vitamin B-12 and folic acid deficiencies are associated with a decrease of red blood cells (called megaloblastic anemia), as well as with other changes in the blood, gastrointestinal tract and cervix. Another sign of B-12, riboflavin, or folic acid deficiency that is more obvious to the individual woman is inflammation of the tongue.

Folic acid (also called folacin) helps the body use proteins, and is a component in the formation of heme (an iron-containing protein in hemoglobin and a necessary part of red blood cells). Folic acid helps the body grow and reproduce appropriately, from a single cell to a fully developed baby. The brain also needs folic acid, and a deficiency can affect mental and emotional health. A deficiency of this vitamin can also cause bleeding gums. Dental researchers have discovered that folic acid supplementation can effectively reduce inflammation and bleeding of the gums if used in a mouthwash solution for just five minutes twice a day.

One of the most exciting pieces of news concerning folic acid supplementation for Pill users is the possibility that this nutrient may reduce their risk of developing cervical cancer. Cervical dysplasia is a change in the cells covering the cervix, the end of the uterus, which juts into the vagina. Cervical displasia is believed to progress to cancer and occurs more often in Pill users. The section on cervical dysplasia in Chapter 2 contains a discussion of folic acid as a treatment for this condition.

Folic acid is easily depleted by poor food choices, injury, bacterial infection, and the use of alcohol. Oral contraceptive users must be especially careful to choose foods rich in this nutrient. Since folic acid is found most profusely in dark-green and leafy vegetables, which seem to be among the foods least attractive to the Americans palate, it is understandable why even non-Pill users are frequently deficient in this nutrient. If you find it difficult to eat greens every day, you may also obtain folic acid from brewer's yeast, whole grains, salmon, and milk. If you're a Pill user, food may not provide enough folic acid for your needs. The World Health Organization has recommended that Pill users supplement with folic acid. So do we.

In theory, taking folic acid without taking B-12 could be dangerous. Folic acid supplementation can cover up symptoms of B-12 deficiency until the body is seriously damaged. However, nutritional doctors would not think of prescribing just one B vitamin, be it B-6 or folic acid, since all the Bs work together. Just be sure to take a B-complex capsule that provides a baseline dose of all the B vitamins.

Vitamin C (Ascorbic Acid)

Researchers suspect that oral contraceptives stimulate the liver to release a certain copper-containing protein called ceruloplasmin, which eradicates vitamin C. Dr. Carl C. Pfeiffer of the Princeton Brain Bio Center in Skillman, New Jersey, reports, "As all research to date has shown, drugs or situations which cause a rise in serum copper demand extra ascorbic acid." The hormones in the Pill may also decrease the absorption of vitamin C, or decrease levels of certain substances that are necessary to the utilization of whatever C is absorbed. No one is sure why Pill users have lower vitamin C levels than nonusers, but research consistently shows that they do.

You can exacerbate this deficiency by continuing to live a stressful lifestyle, and by using coffee, Coke, cigarettes, tetracycline, barbiturates, or even aspirin—all of which sap your body of vitamin C.[6]

In 1979, C. A. B. Clemetson published an interesting theory on the connection between cardiovascular disease and ascorbic acid deficiency. Clemetson noted that the major factors predisposing women to blood clots—the estrogen in oral contraceptives, pregnancy, aging, smoking, infection, trauma, surgery, soft water, and winter—all are associated with decreased ascorbic acid levels. He suggests that blood clots are created when small blood vessels break, owing to a shortage of vitamin C. The body responds to the small hemorrhages by clotting blood, sometimes to excess, creating the critical condition called thrombosis. This, too, is an unproven, but possible, ramification of vitamin C deficiency for Pill users. This theory may explain why birth control pills have been prominently associated with strokes, clots, and cardiovascular disease in young, healthy, and "risk-free" women.

Many doctors are convinced of the benefits of bioflavonoids, which are found in the white pulp beneath the skin of citrus fruits, in black currants and in buckwheat, as a good partner with vitamin C for Pill users, though their effects have not yet been clinically proved. First, certain of the bioflavonoids, specifically rutin, quercetin, and catechin, help pull heavy metals out of the body and thus prevent vitamin C from being eliminated by copper. Since bioflavonoids also strengthen blood vessel walls, many doctors feel that these substances can help vitamin C protect the Pill user from cardiovascular complications of Pill use. Research has demonstrated the benefit of bioflavonoids for women on the Pill who spot-bleed between periods. Bioflavonoids seem to eliminate this breakthrough bleeding.

In addition to supplements and the sources of bioflavonoids mentioned, make sure your daily diet includes some food source of vitamin C, such as strawberries, cantaloupe, green peppers, broccoli, alfalfa sprouts, or citrus fruits.

Vitamin E (Alpha Tocopherol)

Vitamin E is actually a combination of seven substances: alpha, beta, gamma, delta, epsilon, eta, and zeta tocopherol. The alpha form is most biologically active, so, when you buy a vitamin E supplement, make sure it says "alpha tocopherol" on the label rather than mixed, or you will be obtaining less of the most active vitamin E form that your body can use.

The controversy over the value of natural versus synthetic vitamins is probably greater regarding vitamin E than for any other vitamin. Some people insist that natural is better, but at times, this seems more a belief than a scientific observation. The Shute brothers, who pioneered the use of vitamin E for the treatment of cardiovascular disease, miscarriage, and many other conditions, used synthetic alpha tocopherol as soon as it was available. Synthetic E is called dl-alpha tocopherol, whereas a nonsynthetic form is called d-alpha tocopherol. D-alpha tocopherol is found in whole grains, wheat germ, sweet potatoes, leafy vegetables, and cold-pressed oils, especially wheat germ oil and soybean oil (not corn oil).

Vitamin E is a fat-soluble vitamin, and the estrogens in oral contraceptives hamper the liver's ability to metabolize fat-soluble vitamins. One study measured only 40 to 56 percent as much vitamin E in the blood of Pill users as in nonusers. In *Dr. Wilfrid Shute's Vitamin E Book*, Dr. Shute claims that estrogens and alpha tocopherol are antagonistic. He points to the increased risk of hypertension, the fact that women on oral contraceptives have been shown to have 11 times as many dangerous blood clots and twice the incidence of gallbladder disease, coupled with the successful use of vitamin E to improve blood circulation in cases of stroke as strong evidence in favor of this theory. It is also well known in medical circles that birth control pills raise levels of cholesterol, triglycerides, and low-density lipoproteins, all factors that increase the risk of cardiovascular disease. Doctors recognize that even Pill users who don't have measurable deficiencies in vitamin E should take supplements of this vitamin to ward off cardiovascular system problems.

Shute also notes that low thyroid function compounds the danger to women on the Pill, because "estrogen and thyroid extract are antagonistic . . . in people who are low in thyroid activity, cardiovascular damage is increased, both in rate of incidence and in degree."[7] Even mild hypothyroidism, or decreased thyroid function, can lead to increased risk of arteriosclerosis of the brain and other cardiovascular diseases, and Dr. Shute notes that people with hypothyroidism usually have an excess of estrogen and/or a deficiency of vitamin E. If a woman already has high levels of estrogen as a result of hypothyroidism, and then takes oral contraceptives, she is putting herself at greater risk than normal for these life-threatening side effects.

Dr. Broda Barnes, a pioneer in the recognition and treatment of hypothyroidism, recommends that a careful scrutiny of thyroid function should be made in all cases before initiating the Pill, since low thyroid "tends to make for sluggish blood circulation which may then result in a tendency for the blood to coagulate."[8] Please see page 35 for a fuller discussion of hypothyroidism and a simple test you can perform on yourself if you suspect that you are hypothyroid.

As Wilfrid Shute sums up, "Low thyroid, high estrogen, low vitamin E equals a great increase in various cardiovascular problems!" Extra vitamin E and home thyroid testing are good ideas for any Pill taker.

The Minerals

Use of the birth control pill affects levels of a number of minerals, especially manganese, zinc, and copper.

Manganese hasn't been as widely studied as some of the other minerals. Manganese deficiency in oral contraceptive users is inferred by measuring its low level in the breast milk of women who used oral contraceptives before becoming pregnant. Women who have used the Pill prior to conception are advised to take manganese supplements while breast-feeding for the sake of their infant. So it seems logical to suggest that women who are currently on the Pill should take such supplementation for their own sakes.

Zinc and copper are intimately linked in our biochemistry. When zinc levels rise, copper levels drop. When copper levels rise, zinc levels drop. Professor M. K. Horwitt, a professor of biochemistry, and co-workers at St. Louis University investigated the effect of the Pill on the metabolism of blood lipids (fats), vitamins C, A, and E, copper, and the amino acid tryptophan. They found that the most spectacular change resulting from Pill use was in serum copper levels. In fact, they found it possible to judge accurately whether a woman was on the Pill simply by measuring her serum copper level, which was high in all Pill users. (Serum is the watery portion of blood).[9]

The Horwitt study is only one of many that have demonstrated altered trace mineral levels because of oral contraceptive use. Most studies indicate that there is definitely a reduction in zinc and a rise in copper levels. This result may be due to decreased absorption of zinc, increased excretion, a redistribution of minerals within the body, or a decrease in the protein called albumin, which carries zinc in the blood. Low zinc levels certainly are related to the rise in copper caused by the hormones in the Pill. If you also happen to have copper pipes in your home plumbing system, you are magnifying the effect of the Pill-induced abnormal copper-zinc ratio by drinking copper-laced water.

Zinc is important for general body functions, for healing wounds, for proper growth and development of reproductive organs, for proper digestion, and metabolism, and especially for the ability of the body to use B vitamins. It is also crucial for efficient white blood cell function, which fights infection. If you suffer zinc deficiency, your injuries won't heal as well or as fast, you may see stretch marks on your skin and white spots on your fingernails, or you may feel unusually fatigued and lose your appetite and sense of taste.

Besides taking a zinc supplement, you can enhance zinc concentration in your body by eating dark green and leafy vegetables and whole grains, pumpkin seeds, sunflower seeds, brewer's yeast, and seafood, especially oysters.

There are two positive results of oral contraceptive use for body chemistry.

First, oral contraceptives promote an increased absorption of calcium, which is good news to any woman interested in avoiding osteoporosis, the dangerous thinning of bones that often occurs after menopause. Second, since Pill users have less blood loss during menstruation than nonusers, they retain more iron in their bodies. Pill users also have increased iron absorption from their intestines, so it can be assumed that Pill users need less supplemental iron than nonusers.

Daily Supplement Dose Advisory—Contraception

THE IUD

Please see the Daily Supplement Dose Advisory for Painful Menstruation in Chapter 6.

THE PILL

B complex—50 mg of major B vitamins
B-6—50 mg
Folic acid—400–800 mcg
Vitamin C—2,000 mg
Vitamin E—400–800 I.U.
Zinc (elemental)—50 mg
Multimineral—including 1,000 mg calcium and 500 mg magnesium

Chapter Seven:
Infertility

In Brief—Infertility

Symptoms—No pregnancy after a year without using contraception

Signs—In women: low basal body temperature, no ovulation, blocked Fallopian tubes, little cervical mucus, acidic vaginal secretions, failure of fertilized egg to implant (blighted ovum). In men: deformed, immobile, clumped or insufficient sperm.

Cause—In women: incorrect timing of intercourse, hypothyroidism, insufficient body weight, excess body weight, pelvic inflammatory disease, endometriosis, drug use, hormonal imbalance, acidic diet, emotional stress. In men: drugs, disease, varicose vein in testes, toxic chemicals, heat, nutritional deficiencies, emotional stress.

Due to—Ignorance of physiology; improper diet; stress from relationship, work, family pressures; occupational hazards; ignorance of effect of recreational drugs; genetic predisposition.

Solution—For women: surgery, weight gain or loss, stop drug use, supplements, counseling, stress reduction. For men: cold sitzbaths or showers, avoid chemicals, wear boxer shorts, take supplements, reduce stress.

Supplements—Vitamin E, wheat germ oil, vitamin B complex, vitamin C, bioflavonoids, vitamin A, essential fatty acids (safflower oil, borage oil, linseed oil, black currant oil, or evening primrose oil), zinc, multimineral, thyroid hormone.

In order for a baby to be brought successfully to term, conception, implantation, and gestation must take place. Sperm and egg must meet in the woman's Fallopian tube and unite. The small ball of multiplying cells that results must pass through the Fallopian tube and into the uterus, where it must implant on the uterine wall and not in the tube. Once implanted, it must anchor there firmly enough to develop into a growing fetus. Problems leading to infertility can occur anywhere along the way in this process.

About one in six couples is unable to conceive (one in four from ages 35 through 39), and the number of infertile couples has been increasing dramatically ever since the end of World War II.

Although nature isn't always reliable, some couples who thought they were hopelessly infertile are finding out they actually suffer from nutritional deficiencies that are causing reproductive failure. Once they start working with nature and correct their nutritional deficiencies, these couples conceive.

Fertility problems lie with the man in about 40 percent of cases, with the woman about in 50 percent of cases, and with both in about 10 percent of cases. This is a book about women's health, so we include only information that can help women correct any nutritional deficiencies affecting their fertility.

THE RIGHT STUFF

An observant physician in Monroeville, Pennsylvania, suggested an infertile patient stop using her nasal decongestant. She did and became pregnant. The drug had been drying up mucus in her vagina as well as her nose, and sperm hadn't been provided the fluid medium they needed to move up to the egg.

Besides needing moisture, sperm thrive in an alkaline environment. If your vagina is too acidic, the sperm are not going to move with as much vigor. You can measure your body pH with "Nitrazine" tapes, available at a pharmacy, which you insert in your vagina. A color scale on the bottle tells you the meaning of your test results. Lower numbers are acidic, higher are alkaline. The scale on the bottle goes from 4, mildly acidic, to 7.5, mildly alkaline.

Your body works best at a daytime pH of around 5.5, which is slightly acidic; 7.0, the pH of water, is neutral. If your body is too acidic, you may want to change your diet. The foods you eat and how you eat them determine the acid and alkaline balance of the body. Acid fruits such as tomatoes, pineapples, and oranges become alkaline once digested—the acidic portion of the fruit is digested and excreted, but the remaining ash consists of alkaline minerals. Prunes, plums, and cranberries stay acidic throughout the digestive process. Other acid foods include meat, fish, eggs, cheese, seeds, and whole grains. Coffee, alcohol, and other drugs acidify the system. Alkaline foods include milk, fruits, and vegetables. Vitamins and minerals are found in all the above foods, so a diet of exclusively alkaline foods is just as detrimental as a diet of all acidic foods. Balance is the key. Don't forget to eat adequate protein. Protein buffers excess acid in the system, so if you're a haphazard vegetarian (one who doesn't eat meat or fish but who also doesn't pay attention to food combining), start paying attention and each day eat some whole grains with seeds, yogurt or milk with legumes, or other proper protein combination. See *Diet for a Small Planet,* by Frances Moore Lappé, for specifics.

Are you thin? Your weight, or lack of it, can be the cause of a lack of ovulation. Nature doesn't encourage fertility in times of famine or malnutrition. Fat is used by the female body to convert androgens (male hormones produced in small quantities even in females) to estrogens, and affects the biological effectiveness of those estrogens. Even where weight is only 10 to 15 percent below normal the hormones that control ovulation can be lacking.[1]

It is well known that many women athletes stop menstruating, which may be caused by too little body fat. Even athletes who have regular periods may suffer from subtle hormonal irregularities that prevent conception. If you have been controlling your weight through stringent dieting or vigorous exercise, relax some of that self-control. Cut back on your exercise regime, eat more (nutritious foods only), and you may find yourself pregnant before you can say "Nothing fits anymore!"

There is evidence that obese women also are more likely to fail to ovulate than women of normal weight.

Nutritional Imbalances

Health professionals who take a nutritional approach to infertility are not looking for magic in a bottle. They carefully balance the body's biochemistry so every system works efficiently. If nutritional imbalances are the weak link in your reproductive system's chain, some biochemical fine-tuning could set you on your way to family life.

The nutrients that have been implicated in female infertility include essential fatty acids (EFAs), vitamin E, vitamin A, vitamin B-2, vitamin B-6, pantothenic acid, vitamin B-12, folic acid, vitamin C, iron, zinc, magnesium, and tryptophan.

EFAs

Animal studies have pointed to the importance of adequate essential fatty acids for reproductive health. Rats given a diet deficient in fatty acids had trouble reproducing. A high level of polyunsaturated fatty acids, derived from linoleic acid, are found in the Graafian follicles of cattle and pigs. The Graafian follicle is the fluid-filled sac that houses the maturing egg in the ovary. The oil from the seed of the evening primrose flower is especially rich in linoleic acid, as is linseed oil, borage oil, and black currant oil. These oils have been found helpful in a variety of conditions, including eczema, premenstrual syndrome, high cholesterol, and alcoholism. If you are not sure whether you are already getting enough EFAs in your diet, some excess oil won't harm you—and it may be the final step to motherhood.

Vitamin E

Vitamin E has often been associated in the public mind with sexuality, because of animal studies linking E with fertility. Rats fed a diet adequate in every known vitamin except E looked and acted entirely healthy, except for one minor problem—they were sterile. The researchers who originally isolated vitamin E named it tocopherol, from the Greek *tokos,* "birth," and *pherein,* meaning "to carry."

Fatty acids, like all oils and fats, tend to become rancid in the presence of oxygen, a result of oxidation. Scientists are beginning to connect oxidation with aging and the initiation of a variety of degenerative diseases. Vitamin E is a premier antioxidant. It protects the fat portion of all the body cells from becoming rancid and causing biochemical toxicity. This is good news for anybody stressed by polluted air, water, and food. If that sounds familiar, you need more E than those living an unstressed, pollution-free existence (know anyone like that?).

Vitamin E plays an important role in protecting the blood from unnecessary clotting, reducing the oxygen requirement of the heart, helping new blood vessels grow around obstructed capillaries, and helping reduce the contraction of scar tissue. And, by preventing tissue damage to the sex organs, along with the rest of the body, E plays a role in improving fertility.

Vitamins B-12 and B-6

In 1977, Jo Anne Brasal, M.D., of Columbia University told a Nutrition and Human Reproduction conference held at the National Institutes of Health in Bethesda, Maryland, about the use of vitamin B-12 to improve fertility. Brasal reported that some women without apparent medical cause for their conception difficulties are able to conceive within months of receiving vitamin B-12 supplementation.

Dr. Joel T. Hargrove of Columbia, Tennessee, and Dr. Guy E. Abraham of Rolling Hills, California, treated 14 women who had been infertile for from 1½ to 7 years with vitamin B-6. Hargrove and Abraham have published widely on their use of B-6 for premenstrual tension, and these women, too, reported suffering from PMS. The researchers suspected that B-6 might help the women's infertility, because of its effect on the hormone prolactin. Elevated prolactin levels have been found in women who have PMS and who are infertile. It is the hormone that keeps breast milk flowing and the one responsible when there is a lack of menstrual periods or lack of ovulation (the two are not always synonymous) in nursing mothers.

Hargrove and Abraham figured that since high doses of B-6 have been used to stop lactation, thus indicating that it can suppress prolactin, it might help those women conceive whose level of prolactin was excessive. In their study, each woman took enough B-6 for her PMS symptoms to abate, 100 mg to 800 mg per day, depending on the woman. Of the 14 women, 11 became pregnant within six months of B-6 therapy. By the eleventh month, 12 women were pregnant. Hargrove and Abraham also found that before treatment, the women in their study had high levels of estrogen and low progesterone. Progesterone is the female hormone that keeps the uterine lining ready to receive a fertilized egg. After treatment, 7 women's hormone levels were tested. Five of the 7 had significantly higher progesterone levels, a significant change for the infertile women with luteal phase defect.[2]

When the egg erupts from a thinned spot on the ovary wall, the Graafian follicle remains behind and changes into a specialized gland, called the corpus luteum. The "luteal phase" is that period in the menstrual cycle when the corpus luteum secretes progesterone. Women with defective luteal phases don't have adequate progesterone circulating in their body to create a rich, nourishing uterine lining for the fertilized egg. The deficiency may also prevent conception in the first place.

Dr. Richard Taylor of Atlanta, Georgia, uses Optivite® as a treatment for luteal phase defect. This is a nutritional formula developed by Dr. Guy Abraham that contains high doses of B-6 (300 mg), calcium (250 mg), and magnesium (500 mg) (figures are per 12 tablets). The formula for Optivite® provides a 1:2 calcium-magnesium ratio, instead of the usual 2:1 ratio found in other vitamin/mineral products. "In about 90 percent of cases, the hormonal imbalance is due to a nutritional imbalance," Taylor says. The other 10 percent of cases are due to hormonal problems such as thyroid or pituitary deficiencies, or some other even rarer condition.

Taylor points out two common ways that women unknowingly create B-6 deficiencies: coffee and alcohol. Coffee, he says, causes you to excrete B-6 in your urine, and alcohol deactivates the vitamin B-6 that you've managed to keep in your system.

The B 6–progesterone relationship is a perfect example of the ingenious, elegant feedback system of your body. To keep estrogen at an exactly appropriate level, the liver converts excess fat-soluble estrogen into a water-soluble form, which is excreted by the kidneys in your urine. The liver needs vitamin B-6 to perform this conversion. If B-6 is deficient, estrogen builds up in the bloodstream. The ovary gets the message to slow down production of progesterone, and so people with deficient B-6 usually have low progesterone.

"Vitamin B-6 serves as a cofactor in more metabolic functions than any other vitamin," writes the staff of the Princeton Brain Bio Center in Skillman, New Jersey, which develops treatments that use nutrition as a means of healing disease. One of the functions of B-6 is to further the absorption of zinc, another nutrient useful in cases of infertility.

The RDA for B-6 is only 2 mg. There are cases of adverse effects resulting from too much B-6, including tingling in the legs and feet, numbness in the lips and tongue, and impaired sense of touch. These symptoms do not appear all at once, but come on gradually after months of taking hundreds or, in some cases, thousands of milligrams of the vitamin each day. "Too much" is a relative amount, which is obvious from the results of the Abraham-Hargrove study: What created health in one woman was eight times what another woman needed for the same results. However, Dr. Abraham is quick to warn self-dosers that individual B vitamins are never to be taken alone for long, or you will develop deficiencies of other vitamins and minerals. B-6 helps some cases of infertility when included in a total nutritional program, he says. According to Dr. Pfeiffer of the Princeton Brain Bio Center, taking zinc along with B-6 as well as B-complex will eliminate any numbness and tingling. Pfeiffer recommends brewer's yeast as a good source of B-complex vitamins.

If you begin self-dosing with B-6, or *any* supplement, be aware of any unexplained sensations and reactions and cut back what you are taking as a test to see if the reactions disappear. Remain in close contact with a nutritionally experienced health-care provider, who can give advice on your total program and monitor your progress.

The Other Bs

In 1982, the *British Journal of Obstetrics and Gynaecology* published a report on the successful use of folic acid in cases of infertility of 4 to 10 years' duration. Three women given 5 mg of folic acid three times a day became pregnant within 3, 11, and 15 months, respectively. The researchers weren't sure whether the folic acid improved the health of the ovum, the embryo, or the uterine environment in which the fertilized egg implanted and grew.[3]

B-2, or riboflavin, is another member of the B complex that seems to play a role in improved fertility. Lack of riboflavin caused female rats to stop menstruating and, if they were already pregnant, to deliver malformed babies.

Other Bs such as thiamin (B-1) and pantothenic acid are essential for maintaining the pregnancy and for preventing malformations of the growing fetus.

Vitamin A

Inside your Fallopian tubes are minuscule hairlike projections, called cilia, which, along with muscular contractions of the tube wall, move the egg toward the uterus. One of vitamin A's jobs is to keep these tiny fingers moving.

Vitamin A also works with vitamin E to keep cell membranes healthy, influences the creation of proteins in muscles and blood, maintains the mucous membranes of the body, and is generally necessary for reproductive health.

Proper vitamin A absorption requires healthy bile acids. The liver produces bile and also is responsible for handling A and all other fat-soluble vitamins. A healthy liver, then, is one of the prerequisites for proper vitamin A absorption. According to Sheldon C. Deal, a Tucson, Arizona, chiropractor and naturopathic physician, small pustules that look like dried-up whiteheads or dry hair follicles on the back of the arm are an early sign of vitamin A deficiency.[4] Night blindness is a more well-known and striking sign.

When you consume more A than you use, it is stored in your body fat and can build up to toxic levels over time. One of the first signs of vitamin A toxicity is severe headache—a symptom that's hard to miss. Other symptoms include dry, scaly skin, loss of hair and vision problems such as seeing double or blurred vision. If the recommended dose of vitamin A proves too much for your body, cut back. That's the only safe and logical thing to do.

Vitamin C (Ascorbic Acid)

In Japan, gynecologist Masao Igarashi found that vitamin C helped women who failed to ovulate and who were unaided by fertility drugs. When Igarashi gave five such patients vitamin C alone, two began ovulating. A daily dose of 400 mg of C sufficed to induce ovulation and conception for one woman, even though Clomid (clomiphene citrate), a powerful commercially produced fertility drug, used alone had had no effect. When Igarashi combined doses of vitamin C with Clomid, all the women ovulated. In treating other kinds of infertility, he found Clomid more effective when used in conjunction with vitamin C than when used alone.[5]

Magnesium

Magnesium is needed to produce estrogen and progesterone. This is the mineral's direct connection to sterility problems. How do you know if magnesium is what you need? Magnesium deficiency symptoms include nervous irritability, muscle contractions, flatulence and constipation, calcium deposits, impaired blood circulation, falling hair, and broken fingernails.

SUMMARY

Women (and men) who are determined to be parents will abandon greasy fast foods, white-sugar and white-flour products, alcohol, recreational drugs (marijuana lowers sperm count), and caffeine-containing foods and drinks (chocolate, colas, coffee, black tea). They will cut back on their training regimen if they are marathoners, and begin walking if they have been couch potatoes. If no physical obstruction is blocking your tubes or his testicles, a few months of a new diet and supplement program just might change your quiet life forever.

Daily Supplement Dose Advisory—Infertility

Vitamin E—400 to 800 I.U.
Wheat germ oil—1 tablespoon
Vitamin C—2,000 to 5,000 mg
Bioflavonoids—300 mg
Vitamin A—10,000 I.U.
Vitamin B complex—50 to 100 mg of major B vitamins
Essential fatty acids—safflower oil (several teaspoons per day) or evening primrose oil (1,250 mg up to 3 times a day), or borage oil (one capsule per day), or linseed oil (1,250 mg), or black currant oil (as directed on bottle).
Zinc (elemental)—50 mg
Thyroid——as prescribed by physician.

Chapter Eight:

Pregnancy

In Brief—Pregnancy

NORMAL, UNEVENTFUL

Symptoms—No menstrual period, enlarging breasts and abdomen.
Signs—Positive pregnancy test.
Cause—Union of sperm and egg.
Due to—Sexual intercourse or laboratory manipulation.
Solution—Nutritious diet, supplements, exercise, relaxation. It is a self-limiting condition.
Supplements—Folic acid, B-6, iron, strong multivitamin, strong multi-mineral, adequate magnesium, sodium chloride (table salt) to taste. If previous Pill user, add vitamin C.

MORNING SICKNESS

Symptoms—Nausea and vomiting during first trimester.
Signs—Same.
Cause—Possibly excess toxicity or poor digestive function.
Due to—Possibly a deficiency of vitamin B-6, zinc, and/or calcium.
Solution—Supplements, improve diet, attention to food combining, slow movements, protein snacks, balance acid-alkaline relationship, avoid fried foods, drink miso soup, eat yogurt.
Supplements—B-6, zinc, magnesium, phosphoric acid.

TOXEMIA, HIGH BLOOD PRESSURE, EDEMA

Symptoms—Dizziness, headaches, upper abdominal pain, nausea and vomiting, lack of appetite.
Signs—High blood pressure, edema, protein in urine.
Cause—Malnourishment, deficient protein, deficient salt, deficient calcium, deficient magnesium.

Due to—Poor diet choices before and during pregnancy.

Solution—Improve diet, take supplements, consume water and salt to taste.

Supplements—B-6, magnesium, calcium.

VARICOSE VEINS, HEMORRHOIDS

Symptoms—Enlarged, purplish veins on legs or rectum. Hemorrhoids may bleed.

Signs—Same as above.

Cause—Weak smooth muscles in vein walls; poor muscle tone; added pressure on veins.

Due to—Increased blood flow of pregnancy and increased weight of uterus as it pushes downward on abdominal organs and blood vessels; deficiency of nutrients responsible for capillary and connective tissue strength and flexibility.

Solution—Improved diet, supplements, exercise, sitzbaths, eliminate constipation, squat for bowel movements.

Supplements—Calcium, magnesium, vitamin C, bioflavonoids, potassium, vitamin E.

LEG CRAMPS

Symptoms—Pain in the calf.

Signs—Same.

Cause—Lack of calcium, magnesium or potassium, cold muscles forced to work, overexercised muscles.

Due to—Elimination of excess minerals in sweat, dietary deficiency.

Solution—Replace mineral loss by drinking mineral-rich vegetable broths and juices; supplements, improve diet, massage, damp heat.

Supplements—Magnesium, calcium, potassium, hydrochloric acid.

STRETCH MARKS

Symptoms—Reddish lines on breasts, abdomen, and elsewhere that eventually turn white and are slightly depressed below the skin surface.

Signs—Same.

Cause—Lack of sufficient elasticity of stretched skin.

Due to—Lack of protein, lack of vitamins and minerals, genetic predisposition, lack of muscle tone.

Solution—Improved diet, supplements, massage.

Supplements—Zinc, eggs, vitamin E; apply topically fish liver oil or other skin softeners such as cocoa butter, avocado oil, lanolin.

SLEEPLESSNESS

Symptoms—Inability to fall asleep at night.
Signs—Same.
Cause—Excitement, hormones, low blood sugar, hyperthyroidism or worry.
Due to—Eating habits; financial, personal, or anticipated distress; being "wound up" physically and mentally.
Solution—Relaxation exercises, yoga, deep breathing, biofeedback, supplements, change diet, change snack at bedtime, thyroid if prescribed.
Supplement—Magnesium, potassium, zinc, B complex.

Pregnant! With excitement, with awe, you embark upon what will probably be the most taxing, challenging, inspiring and transforming experience of your life. To begin with, you are now responsible for the life of your unborn child. Every morsel you eat, each substance you drink, and even what you breathe, absorb through your skin and, possibly, *think* will affect the development of another human being.

AN UNEVENTFUL PREGNANCY— EVERYONE'S DREAM

If you have planned this pregnancy carefully and were aware of the influence of your diet on the infant's health, you have already stopped using toxic substances such as alcohol, cigarettes, all recreational drugs, food additives and white-sugar and white-flour products. You have been eating foods with the most nutrients, such as whole grains, eggs, seafood, lean meats, soy products, raw or lightly steamed vegetables, fresh fruits in season, fresh nuts, seeds, and sprouts. You've been drinking plenty of filtered water each day (store-bought or obtained through an attachment to your own faucet) and maintained a regular exercise schedule. If you were previously using birth control pills, you have waited several months before becoming pregnant so your body chemistry could rebalance. And you have been taking supplements such as vitamins C and B-6 and folic acid before you got pregnant, to make up for any deficiencies caused by using the Pill. Even a woman who did not use the Pill before becoming pregnant is giving herself and her infant the best chance for an easy, healthy pregnancy and birth if she takes vitamin and mineral supplements.

If it has taken a positive pregnancy test to snap you out of your dietary torpor and focus your attention on nutrition, congratulate yourself for being willing to make the change from eating whatever is convenient or cheap or appealing to eating food that will create a complication-free pregnancy and birth, and an intelligent, alert, and healthy infant. Though the connection between nutrition and infant health has been described in the medical literature for the past 60 years, nutrition hasn't been one of the required courses in medical school. Therefore, it is up to you to gather the information presented here and in books suggested in the bibliography, in order to provide the best opportunity for an easy pregnancy and a healthy baby.

Pregnancy Is Not the Time to Diet

The physiology of the pregnant woman is radically different from when she is not pregnant, and it is wrong to use the same standards of "normalcy" for both conditions. In early pregnancy, nausea can reduce appetite. But once the nausea is gone, the pregnant woman may desire more food than ever before in her life, and may have unusual, extremely strong cravings and aversions. Her blood volume increases, and edema (swelling resulting from excess fluid in connective tissue) is a normal occurrence, especially in the later months. Late in pregnancy, digestion slows down. Muscles relax, including the valve between the stomach and esophagus, so a woman may experience uncomfortable feelings of acidity and heartburn.

A pregnant woman should never consciously attempt to lose weight or even limit her food consumption. It is difficult enough to obtain the recommended levels of essential nutrients when carefully choosing wholesome foods! In numerous studies, pregnant women have been shown to eat less than the RDA of many essential nutrients. The relationship between mother's weight and healthy infants is long established. Underweight mothers produce low birth weight infants and suffer significantly higher rates of cardiac and respiratory problems, anemia, premature rupture of membranes, and endometritis (a serious inflammation of the womb). Their infants also suffer prematurity and low Apgar scores (a measure of the general condition of newborns) more frequently than offspring of women of adequate weight.[1]

While significantly overweight women do have more complications during pregnancy and birth, not all overweight women do, and the complications, such as toxemia, hypertension, and diabetes, are frequently diet-related and may be resolved or controlled by careful manipulation of the woman's nutrient intake. We suspect that both underweight and overweight women have even poorer diets, nutritionally speaking, than the normal-weight woman, and need even more careful attention and education to prevent complications.

Fat is laid down during pregnancy for a purpose—nature doesn't act capriciously when it comes to the survival of offspring. Fat serves the mother as a reserve source of energy during both pregnancy and lactation. Nature gives you just nine months to create a healthy, physically intact child, and a variable number of months thereafter to nurse it, but you have the rest of your life to regain the slim figure of your and your mate's dreams. If your doctor pays more attention to the pounds you gain than to what you are putting in your mouth, we suggest you either look for another obstetrician or educate yourself. Two excellent books are Gail Sforza Brewer's *What*

Every Pregnant Woman Should Know and Betty and Si Kamen's *Total Nutrition During Pregnancy* (see Selected Bibliography).

The Kamens cite medical studies undertaken as early as 1938 indicating that women taking vitamin and mineral supplementation can decrease their risk of premature labor, have fewer children with birth defects, and have the best birth outcome overall for themselves and their infants.[2]

The Supplements Useful in a Normal, Healthy Pregnancy

During pregnancy, your need for many nutrients increases. These include the B complex, vitamin A, vitamin C, iron, vitamin E (especially during the first half of the pregnancy), calcium (especially during the last half of the pregnancy), and other minerals, such as zinc, magnesium, manganese, and chromium.

We recommend a strong multivitamin and a separate multimineral because one tablet cannot contain all the vitamins *and* minerals you need, and still be small enough for a human to swallow. Multivitamin and multimineral supplements will provide you with adequate quantities of these nutrients without your having to buy each one individually, which is hard on the memory, the appetite, and the pocketbook. However they are taken, supplements may be seen as a form of health insurance for a joyful delivery and healthy infant.

If you were to eat a nail, not much of the iron would penetrate into your cells in any useful way. Iron is an inorganic substance and needs help moving from the intestine into the bloodstream and beyond. It is well known that acidic foods, including vitamin C (ascorbic acid) consumed along with iron gives this mineral an added boost along the biochemical path from gut to blood. Attaching the iron to an amino acid, a form called "chelated iron," is another way to improve this product's absorption. Some of the most easily absorbed forms of iron are iron aspartate (attached to aspartic acid), iron peptonate (attached to a peptone, a short-chain amino acid), and iron citrate (attached to citric acid).

We recommend iron citrate, an unusual but highly absorbable form that does not turn your stools black, give you an egg-on-the-breath odor, upset your stomach, or cause constipation, as does iron sulphate, the form most common in the average iron pill. Thorne Research, Inc., of Seattle, manufactures an excellent iron citrate. The company sells only to medical professionals, so you can ask your obstetrician to order it for you. Thorne's address is 610 Andover Park East, Seattle, Washington 98188; (800) 228-1966 (206) 575-0777.

MORNING SICKNESS

No one is sure why some women are nauseated during the first few months of their pregnancies and others aren't; but some researchers believe the problem is actually a positive sign that the body contains higher levels of hormones needed to maintain the pregnancy. This was the conclusion of a study of over 9,098 pregnancies sponsored by the National Institute of Child Health and Human Development. Women who vomited during their first trimester had nearly a third lower rate of miscarriages and stillbirths and a 17 percent lower rate of premature delivery than those who didn't.[3]

When you are in the throes of nausea, promises of a better chance at a healthy birth may seem a distant reward. You want relief now! But when your baby is born, the nausea that overwhelms you daily right now will be a distant memory, while the baby in your arms will be very real. Don't take a chance with that precious body inside you by taking any kind of drug, be it prescribed, over-the-counter, or left over from a friend or relative's pregnancy, to counter your nausea.

Benedectin, an antinausea medication manufactured by Merrell Dow Pharmaceutical, was clouded in controversy after it was charged that this supposedly harmless medication caused limb deformities in infants, as well as other congenital malformations such as pyloric stenosis, an abnormal closing of the valve between the stomach and the small intestine, which necessitates surgery on the newborn. The manufacturers withdrew the drug from the market after they were forced by a lawsuit to pay $750,000 to the family of a little girl who was born with a deformed arm and hand.

Relief of nausea may be found outside the realm of pharmaceuticals, in simple changes in and additions to your daily menu. One mother relates, "Fifteen years ago, during my first pregnancy, I had no idea that my four miserable months of morning sickness had anything to do with my breakfasts of pork sausages and scrambled eggs, lunches of buttered noodles, and suppers of frozen chicken pot pies. I read the standard advice to eat a few crackers each morning and faithfully ate four Saltines each morning before cooking my sausages."

During her second pregnancy many years later, she discovered that a morning cup of miso soup not only eliminated her nausea, but also improved her energy. Miso paste is made from fermented soybeans, and is mixed with boiled water for a nourishing broth that not only offers a source of protein, but contains lactobacillus bacteria, which aids in digestion. Miso can be purchased at a health-food store. Yogurt is another source of lactobacillus, if you purchase a brand that states on the carton it contains active cultures.

Other digestive tract soothers include carbonated water and raspberry leaf, peppermint, or spearmint tea—*not* black tea, which contains caffeine. In addition, you may want to use a digestive enhancer that includes betaine hydrochloric acid (for better protein digestion), and pancreatic enzymes (for better carbohydrate digestion). Using these digestive aids with each meal can make a big difference if you suffer gas, bloating, and general indigestion after meals.

Avoiding fried, fatty foods as well as junk foods loaded with sugar, white flour, and chemicals also has been found to help relieve the discomfort of morning sickness.

Excess acidity in your stomach may be causing the morning sickness. Coffee, which causes your stomach to release acid, should be avoided.

Other methods to avoid acidity include not eating for several hours before going to bed and avoiding overconsumption of acid-forming foods. Even healthy foods like some fruits and whole grains can increase acidity. Fruit is acidic on the way through the digestive tract, though it becomes alkaline at the end of digestion. The only fruits that remain acidic throughout digestion are cranberries, prunes, and plums. If you are eating lots of prunes to counter constipation, this may be one cause of your nausea.

Become aware of the possible connection between food combinations and your nausea. Combining fruits with protein-rich foods—such as yogurt with fruit mixed in, or eggs and orange juice—could cause nausea. See what happens if you leave at least a half hour between eating fruit and other food. You may want to avoid orange and grapefruit juice entirely. These juices are concentrations of sugar, which makes your pancreas work harder to get the sugar out of the bloodstream, and citric acid, which leaches calcium from your body. It's better to eat a whole orange or grapefruit—then you'll get the benefit of the fruit's fibers and of the bioflavonoids in the rind.

Foods that stay acidic throughout the digestive process include whole grains, meat, fish, eggs, and dairy products. Although you need protein during pregnancy, be sure your protein sources are extra lean, and avoid sauces, or any oily, buttery, fatty foods. Keep lean, high-protein finger foods available in the refrigerator for easy snacking, such as a hard-boiled egg, a slice of turkey, or a piece of roasted or broiled chicken. Protein snacks, even in the middle of the night, have helped some women relieve their nausea. Or maybe you will feel better if you eat protein foods earlier in the day, and eat the more alkaline foods (vegetables, or, separately, fruits) at night. That way, your stomach will not be stimulated during the night to produce the quantity of hydrochloric acid needed to digest proteins.

Calcium, magnesium, sodium, and potassium are the alkaline-forming minerals. If your body is too acidic, supplementation with any of these minerals may help rebalance your biochemistry. It is interesting to note that magnesium and calcium are both smooth-muscle relaxants. One theory of morning sickness is that it occurs when toxins eliminated by the fetus cause smooth muscle of the stomach and gall bladder ducts to constrict, slowing down liver and bile function.

Besides mineral supplementation, you may find relief from morning sickness by drinking a solution of liquid Phosfood. Phosfood is the brand name of phosphoric acid manufactured by Standard Process Laboratories, Inc., of Milwaukee. One health-care provider has found that 50 drops of Phosfood in a glass of water can provide instant relief. If you are unable to find a store selling Phosfood try Emetrol, manufactured by Adria of Columbus, Ohio. Emetrol is a combination of phosphoric acid and two sugars, dextrose and levulose, and is available from your local pharmacy. One note of caution: If you frequently suffer from canker sores, the acidity of the phosphoric acid may cause them to reappear.

Probably the nutritional supplement most often used in cases of morning sickness is vitamin B-6. B-6 is needed by rapidly growing tissues, such as those of the fetus. It also helps the mother's body eliminate harmful environmental pollutants as well as the metabolic waste discharged by the fetus. This vitamin has an antagonistic relationship to estrogen, meaning that the more estrogen is present in the body, the more B-6 is needed. Estrogen levels are high during pregnancy. Unfortunately, it is also one of the vitamins most frequently lacking in a pregnant woman's diet. In one study, by the thirty-seventh week of pregnancy only 3 percent of the subjects' daily food intakes contained even the RDA of just 2.6 mg for pregnant women.[4] Women who have taken oral contraceptives for many years before becoming pregnant are at special risk of vitamin B-6 deficiency. Long-term Pill users have been found to have significantly lower levels of B-6 during pregnancy, at delivery, and in their milk, compared to short-term (up to 30 months) users or non-users.[5]

There have been a number of conflicting conclusions in studies using B-6 for morning sickness. One study indicated that there was no clear-cut connection between B-6 deficiency and morning sickness while another found that women with nausea and vomiting had a deficiency of pyridoxal phosphate, the most important form of vitamin B-6. Whether or not there is a measurable deficiency of B-6 in those women who suffer morning sickness, the bottom line is that B-6 supplementation works well for some women, and not for others. Of course, both the dosage of B-6 and other food taken with it may affect its value.

Dr. Carl C. Pfeiffer, director of the Princeton Brain Bio Center in Skillman, New Jersey, and a respected researcher in nutritional medicine, suggests that B-6 taken along with zinc is more effective than B-6 taken alone.[6] If B-6 doesn't work for you, it may be that you aren't taking enough. Although the RDA is only 2.6 mg for pregnant women, nutrition-minded physicians have commonly prescribed as much as 100 mg a day without any discernible negative effects—in fact, the blood of infants born to these women benefited by having a greater ability to take up oxygen, compared to unsupplemented controls. It makes sense to begin with a much lower dose, and see if it works. If not, you can always increase your dosage step by step. If you use 100 mg a day and are still nauseated, add one or more of our suggested treatments against nausea until it disappears, then cut back one by one on the treatments you're using, until you find the minimum treatment that eliminates your nausea.

Magnesium is our final suggestion for nutritional treatment of morning sickness. Eat foods such as almonds and other nuts, legumes (peanuts, lentils, peas and beans), grains, and dark-green vegetables, or take magnesium in supplement form. Not only is nausea a possible sign of magnesium deficiency, but persistent vomiting is one cause of this deficiency, as is chronic stress. When you have too little magnesium, your muscles have difficulty relaxing. Swollen gums, loss of hair, muscle tremors, gastrointestinal distress, and lack of appetite are other symptoms of magnesium deficiency. If that strong multimineral supplement we suggested already doesn't do the trick, consult with a nutrition-minded physician on an appropriate dose of magnesium chelate. We recommend using the chelated form of minerals, for better absorption.

Regardless of what books, friends, or physicians tell you, your stomach is responding to this pregnancy in your own, unique way. Do try to experience all of these alternative treatments before you throw up your hands, along with your lunch, and decide that "nothing works."

TOXEMIA, HIGH BLOOD PRESSURE, EDEMA

Toxemia (Preeclampsia)

If you experience significant weight gain, along with edema, high blood pressure, and measurable protein in your urine, you have a problem that must be treated immediately to protect your life. The problem is called toxemia, or preeclampsia; additional symptoms may be a lack of appetite, nausea and vomiting, dizziness, headache, and upper abdominal pain.

Preeclampsia is the early stage of the full-blown condition called eclampsia, which includes such severe effects of the above-mentioned symptoms that the mother goes into convulsions and even into a coma. It is one of the major causes of maternal death, so early treatment is crucial. Catching these early signs of toxemia as soon as they arise is the main reason for prenatal care. This is why you are asked to step on the scales, provide a urine specimen, and have your blood pressure read whenever you visit your obstetrician during your pregnancy.

For more than half a century, observant clinicians have noticed that toxemia was *not* caused by obesity, first-time or multiple pregnancy, nor by genetics, race, or social class per se, as was earlier thought. Instead, they realized that toxemia was caused by a lack of protein in the diet.

Dr. Thomas H. Brewer, a crusader for better nutrition during pregnancy, describes the condition he calls "metabolic toxemia of late pregnancy" a disease of the liver that is caused by malnutrition. High blood pressure results from low blood volume and poor liver function. Edema develops when the blood is deficient in protein, especially albumin; this deficiency causes fluid to escape from the bloodstream into surrounding tissues.

Brewer berates doctors and nurses who restrict pregnant women's salt and calorie intake and give them diuretics, when they actually need greater blood volume, not less. He calls this treatment an "irrational approach to management of the pregnant woman's diet" that causes so much damage that it has been termed Thalidomide II. In contrast, he cites the impressive statistics collected by five different physicians (including himself) whose work spans 35 years and three continents and who, collectively, have supervised 26,250 pregnancies. They have seen *no* cases of the later stage of toxemia called eclampsia; their secret weapon was high-quality diets, salted food to taste, and plenty of water.[7] Brewer reports research done in London comparing a thousand women who ate a low-salt diet to those eating a high-salt diet.[8]

There are several other important supplements for cases of toxemia. Vitamin B-6 is a natural diuretic. Dr. Jonathan Wright of Kent, Washington, who teaches physicians how to use nutrition in their practices, credits Dr. John M. Ellis with originating an effective treatment combining vitamin B-6 (pyridoxine) with magnesium. Wright notes that magnesium is a necessary partner of B-6 in many important biochemical reactions, even in the nonpregnant body. Calcium is another supplement that may reduce toxemia. In one study, only 440 mg of calcium per day reduced the incidence of toxemia by two thirds.

Eat lean meat and fish, eggs, legumes, whole grains, dairy products (if you aren't allergic to milk), lightly steamed dark-green and leafy vegetables, and a variety of other vegetables and fruits. Be sure that your snacks are also nutritious, such as a hard boiled egg, a piece of chicken, or cheese. If you are a vegetarian, it is particularly important to pay attention to obtaining adequate protein. Carrot sticks and apples do not a healthy baby make. Be sure you are combining grains and seeds, corn and beans, and tofu and grains to get the complete proteins your body and your baby's body need. If you would like more specific advice on combining foods to increase your protein intake, consult Frances Moore Lappé's classic *Diet for a Small Planet.*

High Blood Pressure

Is your blood pressure above 140/90? Or has it been rising significantly over the past few weeks? This is a red flag that will cause your obstetrician concern.

Salt restriction has been the immediate response of standard medical practitioners to high blood pressure. The body's self-correcting mechanism reacts to a lack of salt by releasing a hormone, renin, which starts a hormonal chain reaction, ending in constriction of blood vessels and an even greater increase in blood pressure. Thirty years ago, Dr. Margaret Robinson divided the poor women who came to a public clinic in London into two equal groups and requested that one group reduce their salt intake and the other half increase it. The results: "The low-salt group had nearly three times more damaged placentas, two and a half times more toxemia, and twice the number of infant deaths."[9] In contrast, the high-salt group had fewer complications during pregnancy and delivery. Usually animal experiments precede human ones, but in this case Robinson's work inspired a Pennsylvania State University nutritionist named Ruth Pike to try out the salt study on rats. Pike found that the "no-salt" rats suffered damage to their kidneys and adrenal glands, and the "no-salt" offspring were of lower than normal birth weight. If salt was given to the rat mothers even just three days before delivery, these pathological changes were reversed.

So you see why adequate sodium chloride (table salt) is one of the primary supplements in cases of high blood pressure and hypertension during pregnancy. Have you desired salty foods, but controlled your craving for fear of the consequences? It's time to trust your body. Your taste buds and appetite centers are designed for your survival. When your body needs salt, you'll wish your food were a bit more salty.

Other useful remedies and preventive treatments for high blood pressure using nutrition and nutritional supplements are discussed under Toxemia, above. Since none are prescription products, and all are within your ability to use on your own, there is really no reason for delay!

Edema

If you took a watertight rag doll and pumped 40 percent more filling into it today than it had yesterday, what would it look like? Puffy? You bet! That's you, with 40 percent more blood than you carried around inside before pregnancy. No wonder your hands and feet swell during the last trimester, especially if you are unlucky enough to be pregnant during hot summer months.

Edema is a danger sign, possibly indicating toxemia, if accompanied by high blood pressure and protein in the urine. Whether you have these serious signs or not, do *not* take a diuretic. Your organs need fluids to keep functioning. What the body desperately needs is to lure the fluid out of the body cells and back into the blood. Dr. Tom Brewer in 1960 gave women suffering toxemia human serum albumin, a large protein normally found in blood. Their swelling diminished and their urinary output increased.

Edema *without* protein in the urine or high blood pressure is a normal condition during pregnancy, albeit an uncomfortable one. If you don't have protein in your urine (which you can discover yourself, using a simple dip-stick purchased at any pharmacy), then try some of these common-sense suggestions to relieve your discomfort.

Keep your feet up as much as possible. Put a box next to the sink, so you can raise one leg as you work, which will help with backaches, too. Place a stool next to your typing table or under your desk, so you can raise your feet during your hours on the job. Don't stand at the water cooler or sit in a restaurant during breaks and lunch—get those feet up up up at every opportunity. It may mean inviting a special friend to join you for lunch on the grass in a corner of the lot, or sitting where you can raise your legs on a chair in the cafeteria.

When you sleep, put pillows beneath your knees and ankles to keep the blood from pooling in your extremities overnight. Keep tight clothing, including knee-high stockings, socks, and tight long pants in your drawer until after delivery. This doesn't apply to support hose, which you may decide to try if you also suffer from varicose veins (see below).

Vitamin B-6 and magnesium can help your body eliminate the unwanted swelling, as detailed in the "Toxemia" section, above.

VARICOSE VEINS AND HEMORRHOIDS

Weak blood vessel walls tend to balloon outward with the increased pressure of the pregnant woman's uterus on abdominal organs and veins and with increased blood volume. However, varicose veins in the legs or in the anus and rectum (hemorrhoids) are a sign of something else going on in your body besides pregnancy. Varicose veins may signal a need for potassium, vitamin C, bioflavonoids, calcium, or magnesium and/or vitamin E. Although hemorrhoid treatments are available over the counter, don't use them. Treat the cause, not the end result of your body's condition, for lasting results that are safe for your developing child.

Vitamin C is necessary for the synthesis of collagen, a protein that provides the basics from which the body's tiniest blood vessels, the capillaries, are made. Bioflavonoids are a group of substances found in the white rind of citrus fruits, as well as in grapes, plums, apricots, buckwheat, cherries, and blackberries. Bioflavonoids help vitamin C move from bloodstream to organs where it is needed, help protect vitamin C from destruction, and they also keep the walls of capillaries strong. Although scientific validation for the effectiveness of consuming bioflavonoids to improve capillary fragility is controversial, we suggest this treatment as one alternative you can try, if you suffer from hemorrhoids. It seems prudent to take a vitamin C supplement that includes bioflavonoids as a treatment for this uncomfortable and embarrassing condition.

Potassium, calcium, and magnesium are other nutrients important to muscle health.

If you are beginning to notice varicose veins developing in your legs, stronger muscles will help strengthen your veins and prevent further trouble. Swimming, walking, bicycling, or even simply doing isometric exercises in your home, will improve the tone of the muscles surrounding the veins, and reduce the tendency of blood to pool in unsightly and uncomfortable gnarls.

Don't sit on the toilet for a second longer than you have to! In many other societies, women squat to make bowel movements, and this is a far more physiologically appropriate position to stimulate bowel action as well as to avoid the unhealthy pressure on blood vessels caused by a hard toilet seat. If you can manage it, you may want to put two toddler one-step stools by the toilet and stand on them, resting your weight on your thighs as you defecate. Don't sit down on the toilet until you are ready to eliminate. This will help your hemorrhoids and any constipation you may have.

When you sit in a chair, don't cross your legs. If you must cross them, do so at the ankle, not the knee. And elevate your legs as much as possible, day and night. It's easier for the heart to pump blood downward than for the muscles to squeeze the blood back up your legs.

Sitzbaths, in which you sit in enough water to cover your buttocks and hold your hands and feet out of the water, are also used to stimulate the movement of blood. If you use two small tubs, such as two baby baths, you can fill one with hot water and one with cold water. Sit in the hot water a few minutes, then switch to the cold water for a few seconds, then back to the hot. Or, if you don't want to go through all that, simply sit in hot or cold water a few times a day. Warm water may feel more pleasant, but cold water will contract the muscles surrounding the protruding veins and help shrink them.

One cause of hemorrhoids is constipation. Review your diet. Are you drinking a glass of water frequently during the day? Are you eating whole-grain cereals, pancakes, and muffins for breakfast, or donuts or white-flour pancakes, which may be sitting in your intestines in a stodgy lump? When was the last time you downed a sweet potato, raw fruits, or a salad with numerous colorful vegetables in it? If you don't provide your body with a fiber broom, it can't houseclean.

Veins, like arteries, have smooth muscles around them. Ray Peat, a Eugene, Oregon, biologist who specializes in physiology and nutrition, points out that varicosities are due to loss of muscle tone rather than weak blood vessel valves.[10] A loss of muscle tone, suggests Peat, allows the vein to widen so that the valve cannot reach across it to do its job of closing the vessel. If Peat's theory is correct, then improving muscle tone of those smooth muscles will help the vessel return to its normal size, and the valve will do its job of relieving the varicosity.

LEG CRAMPS

Cramps? Think minerals! Leg cramps can be caused by a lack of any one of several different minerals. During pregnancy, one very common cause of leg cramps is a lack of calcium. If this is the cause of your cramps, you may also be suffering bone loss around your teeth, and painful intestinal spasms as well. You can thank the cramps for warning you that your infant may be taking so much of your calcium, that you must replenish your supply fast and now. Or, you might have caused the deficiency yourself, by drinking an excess of phosphorus-rich soda pop; the greater the level of phosphorus, the lower the level of calcium available to be used by the body. Another reason for calcium deficiency is poor digestion, caused by hydrochloric acid deficiency. Without adequate hydrochloric acid, you cannot move the calcium you eat from your intestines into the bloodstream. Since magnesium and calcium are a team, you are also going to need greater levels of magnesium when you increase your daily calcium intake.

Dr. Ross Trattler, a naturopathic physician in Hilo, Hawaii, gives patients with leg cramps fresh fruit, vegetable juices, and vegetable soups to increase mineral levels.[11] For the broths, why not drop in some soup bones, along with a tablespoon of cider vingar? According to *Natural Remedies for Pregnancy Discomforts* (see the Selected Bibliography), this is a traditional Chinese method for enhancing the nourishment of soups; the vinegar draws the calcium out of the soup bones. Tofu, sesame seeds, broccoli, oysters, sardines, almonds, collard greens, black-eyed peas, and blackstrap molasses are some other rich sources of calcium, along with dairy products.

And don't forget heat and massage. Soak cramped legs in warm water and rub them. Stretch your leg muscles by pointing your toes toward your knees. And take calcium and magnesium supplements immediately.

STRETCH MARKS

Some say there is little that can be done to avoid the white streaks that occur in skin stretched beyond its capacity to rebound. Once the damage is done, they say, it can't be undone. A scar remains a scar. Maybe, and maybe not.

Skin is made to stretch, thanks to the elastin and collagen fibers within it. These fibers do have their limit, and when that limit is reached, the fibers rupture. That limit varies from person to person and may be determined in part by diet.

The magnificent belly of late pregnancy taps the skin's elasticity "to the max," and pregnancy and stretch marks frequently go hand in hand. It's a good idea to think ahead and do what you can to prevent stretch marks from occurring. Malnourished individuals have less elastic skin, so be careful to maintain good nutrition before and during pregnancy. That means making sure your daily diet contains plenty of protein, complex carbohydrates, vitamins, minerals, and fatty acids (for example, those found in sunflower seeds and vegetable oils).

Zinc can also help. The zinc can be taken orally, or can also be effective when rubbed onto the skin directly. Physicians have used zinc oxide to speed up the healing of injured skin, and you can use it to shrink the damaged, stretched tissues of your abdomen and breasts. Or, use another lubricating and nourishing substance, such as a fish liver oil (rich in vitamins A and D), lanolin, castor oil, or vitamin E. Some women swear by cocoa butter.

Ray Peat reports that a number of pregnant women who consumed several egg custards a week, so that they were eating about four eggs a week, watched their stretch marks disappear during pregnancy. If nothing else, it's a delicious experiment, as long as you like eggs and are not allergic to them.

Several sources on stretch marks mention obesity as a factor. Weight gain alone, however, is not an adequate explanation, since plenty of pregnant women whose bellies extend far into space give birth and then regain their same old flat, smooth, blemish-free abdomens within months. So we tend to believe that the phenomenon has much to do with a mix of nutrition and genetics.

If you're eating well and taking nutrients and still those miserable marks appear, there is something else you can do besides blame the throw of your genetic dice. Stretch marks are basically scars, and treatment of scars falls within the province of vitamin E. Try nightly rubbings of the oil for several months, as visible improvement doesn't happen overnight.

One last suggestion—massage! If stretch marks threaten, moisten your fingertips with glycerin, which is available in any drugstore, or a light oil (you can use vegetable oil or buy avocado or almond oil at a health-food store) and rub your abdomen to and fro. Up to 15 minutes of massage daily during pregnancy can help enhance elasticity and prevent stretch marks.

SLEEPLESSNESS

Wendy was seven months pregnant and so desperate for sleep that she was willing to try anything. Her doctor prescribed an antihistamine with sedative side effects, which she took, to no avail. She heard about wonders of warm milk at bedtime, but that didn't work, either. She found a reference to insomnia in *Nutrition for Women,* by Ray Peat, which suggested magnesium, potassium, the B complex, and zinc as well as the old standby, tryptophan. Peat also emphasized the importance of maintaining good blood sugar levels, to avoid the secretion of the alertness hormone, adrenaline, which occurs when blood sugar levels are low.[12] Sources of magnesium, potassium and zinc include bananas and sunflower seeds. Sleep followed for Wendy after she started eating these foods at bedtime.

Bananas do double duty, as a form of complex carbohydrate to keep blood sugar adequate and also as a source of potassium. Wendy had gone to a health food store searching for pumpkin seeds, which are high in zinc, but the store had only salted pumpkin seeds, so she bought sunflower seeds instead. These seeds are also high in protein, potassium, and calcium, making them an excellent choice. Oatmeal would also be a good choice as an evening night-cap, providing magnesium and a good complex carbohydrate to maintain blood sugar. Brewer's yeast is one of the finest all-around nutritional supplements, containing 16 amino acids, 14 minerals and 17 vitamins, including chromium, to keep blood sugar at proper levels, and a rich supply of vitamin B complex for a happy nervous system. Taken before bedtime, it may help solve your sleeplessness problem. In addition, brewer's yeast happens to be an antidote for constipation. The yeast has a taste that some people love and some hate. Luckily, it comes in tablet form as well, so even nose wrinklers can benefit from its nutritional gifts.

Unlike drugs, alcohol, or a knock on the head, nutritional sleeping potions nourished Wendy and her infant while curing her insomnia. You may also want to try other alternatives: deep, rhythmic breathing, either lying in bed or sitting comfortably in a chair; meditation; some simple yoga positions or stretches; taking a walk; or writing in a journal.

And there is one other possible cause of sleeplessness: that all-around culprit, hypothyroidism. Low thyroid hormone is a cause of low blood sugar, and low blood sugar is a cause of sleeplessness. If you were bordering on low thyroid function before pregnancy and did nothing about it, you may want to check back with your physician to see if you should be taking thyroid now to bring your hormone level to normal.

Your insomnia may be due to worry, stress, and unresolved problems carried over to the bedroom. There is so much to think about, with the imminent addition to your family inspiring both dreams and anxieties about the changes to come. Do everything you can to relax naturally. Listen to soft, serene music, or you may want to see a biofeedback technician for some training in self-relaxation. You don't have to stand for sleeplessness another night.

Daily Supplement Dose Advisory—Pregnancy

NORMAL

Folic acid—800 mcg (1st trimester) 400 mcg (2nd trimester)
Vitamin B-6—50–100 mg.

Multivitamin—should contain at least 50 mg B-6
Iron—32 mg
Multimineral—should have at least 32 mg iron, 800 mg calcium, and 400
    mg magnesium
Table salt—to taste
Vitamin C (for ex–Pill users)—1,000 mg

MORNING SICKNESS

Vitamin B-6—50 mg
Zinc—25 mg of elemental zinc
Magnesium—800 mg
Phosphoric acid—"orthophosphoric acid" taken as directed on container

TOXEMIA, HIGH BLOOD PRESSURE, AND EDEMA

Vitamin B-6—100 mg
Magnesium—800 mg
Calcium—800–1,200 mg
Table salt—to taste

VARICOSE VEINS AND HEMORRHOIDS

Calcium—1,000 mg
Magnesium—500 mg
Vitamin C—1,000 mg
Bioflavonoids—300 mg of quercitin in combination with other bioflavo-
    noids
Potassium—99 mg
Vitamin E—400 I.U.

LEG CRAMPS

Magnesium—500 mg
Calcium—1,000 mg
Potassium—99 mg
Betaine hydrochloride—as directed on bottle
Folic acid—800 mcg

STRETCH MARKS

Zinc—25 mg of elemental zinc
Eggs—According to appetite, but try 4 per week
Vitamin E—800 I.U. orally and applied to skin
Fish liver oil, cocoa butter, avocado oil, lanolin—Apply to skin

SLEEPLESSNESS

Magnesium—800 mg
Potassium—99 mg

Zinc—25 mg of elemental zinc

Vitamin B complex (or brewer's yeast)—look for at least 50 mg of major
B vitamins

Tryptophan—from 500–3,000 mg, depending on individual need

PREVENTING BIRTH DEFECTS

Multivitamin

Multimineral—see "Normal" above

Folic acid—1 mg (no history of spina bifida); 4 mg (previously delivered
a child with spina bifida)

Vitamin C—2,000 mg

B complex—containing at least 500 mcg of B-12

Amino acids—500 mg of cysteine (in cases of heavy metal toxicity)

Chapter Nine:
Miscarriage

In Brief—Miscarriage

Symptoms—Bleeding, passing large clots of blood and tissue, painful cramping.

Signs—Dilatation of the cervix and inflammation in the region of implantation, passage of embryo and placenta.

Caused by—Defective ovum, maternal disease, hormonal imbalance, malnutrition and specific nutrient deficiencies, immune system factors, drugs, toxicity, uterine defects, trauma, IUD.

Due to—Chance, genetic outcome, environmental pollutants, viruses, antibiotics, hypertension, diabetes, syphilis, hypothyroidism, deficient diet, excess vitamin antagonists such as coffee and alcohol, congenital abnormalities of the uterus, fibroid tumors, car accident, other trauma, nutrient deficiencies.

Solutions—Detoxify body of pollutants, heal from disease before another conception occurs, take supplements, improve diet.

Supplements—Thyroid, zinc, vitamin B-6, B complex, folic acid, magnesium, vitamin E, vitamin C, bioflavonoids, tryptophan.

Every year more than one in 10 women miscarry. If you ask your friends, you'll be amazed to discover just how common miscarriage is. Probably some of your own relatives and associates have miscarried between pregnancies. Those are the known cases. Many, many other women miscarry and never know they were pregnant. In these cases, the menstrual flow might be more painful, with more clots than normal, but still nothing alarming enough to warrant seeing a doctor.

WHEN SUPPLEMENTS CAN HELP
Thyroid

Dr. Broda Barnes describes one of his miscarriage-prone patients in *Hypothyroidism: The Unsuspected Illness.* She was the wife of a psychiatrist and had three children, although she'd been pregnant seven times. Reviewing her health history, Barnes and the patient found that she had had her babies during the times when she took thyroid, but as soon as she felt well, she had discontinued the medication. The miscarriages occurred during the times she had stopped taking thyroid.

Although hypothyroidism is only one of many causes for miscarriage, if you are low in thyroid hormone, it could easily be the cause of yours. Please read the discussion of hypothyroidism on page 35 for more complete advice about your options.

Progesterone

Each month, the egg develops inside the ovary within a little sack called a follicle. At ovulation time the follicle and the wall of the ovary rupture and discharge an egg. The follicle transforms itself into a gland called the corpus luteum ("yellow body" in Latin), which is the major source of the progesterone that is needed for the first four crucial months of pregnancy. When the placenta, which separates the fetal blood system from the mother's, is fully formed, it takes over the secretion of progesterone and the other hormones needed to keep the pregnancy going.

Some women have what is known as a "luteal phase defect," which means that their corpus luteum is not producing enough hormones, particularly progesterone, to maintain the pregnancy, and miscarriage results. Although the immediate solution seems to be to give the woman more progesterone, a physician who is looking at the larger picture will ask why the woman's body is producing so little of this hormone, and will treat the cause rather than the symptom.

Often, the cause of progesterone deficiency is nutritional. Atlanta, Georgia, obstetrician-gynecologist Richard Taylor uses Optivite® (manufactured by Optimox, of Torrance, California), a multivitamin with a high dose of B-6 and magnesium in its formula, to protect the pregnancy. These nutrients help the liver rid the body of extra estrogen, and as estrogen levels fall, progesterone levels rise.

Vitamin B-6

Some of the pioneering work of Southern California gynecologist-researcher Guy Abraham (formulator of the Optivite® Supplement) focused on the importance of vitamin B-6 in the liver. This vitamin helps the liver convert the fat-soluble form of estrogen to a water-soluble form, which can be excreted by the kidneys in the urine. A B-6 deficiency permits estrogens to build up in the system, and the ovary responds by slowing down its production of progesterone. That is why women with low B-6 levels can be chronic aborters, explains Dr. Taylor, who uses Optivite ® as a basic nutritional program for many hormone-related gynecological conditions.

Taylor points out that both alcohol and caffeine deplete the body of B-6— alcohol by deactivating the vitamin, and caffeine by increasing the excretion of B-6 in the urine.

Zinc

A pregnancy is a complicated interaction of many different hormones and body systems. One system not often discussed is the immune system. A woman must make antibodies to alert her own body to the presence of the developing fetus, which otherwise would be identified as a foreign invader and eliminated. Zinc is a crucial factor in the proper functioning of the immune system. Zinc deficiency can cause any number of defects in this intricate and important defense system, including miscarriage.[1] Animal studies have also shown that diets low in zinc cause miscarriages, as well as abnormal fetuses. Zinc is necessary for folic acid to be properly absorbed, and there is clear evidence that folic acid is an essential nutrient for a successful and healthy pregnancy. Do you know any families with a string of girl children punctuated by a string of miscarriages in between? The mother may possibly be zinc deficient. Dr. Carl Pfeiffer suggests that since male babies need more zinc than females, a pregnant woman deficient in this mineral would be more likely to miscarry a male fetus.

Dr. Pfeiffer explains that zinc is needed to transform vitamin B-6 from its inactive to its active form in the body. Zinc and B-6 work well together, because B-6 helps zinc absorption. A woman preparing her body for the nutritional challenge of pregnancy should take both B-6 and zinc.

B Complex

The total B complex includes B-1 (thiamin), B-2 (riboflavin), B-3 (niacin), B-6 (pyridoxine), B-12 (cobalamin), folic acid, pantothenic acid, biotin, inositol, and choline. Each B vitamin has its own role in body function, centered on the nervous system. Since nerves bring messages to all the organs and stimulate glands to secrete their important biochemicals, the body communication system can break down when there is a deficiency of B vitamins.

This group of vitamins works together synergystically. Each has its specific tasks, but if you take a disproportionately large dose of one B vitamin, after a few weeks the body will begin to complain with myriad distress symptoms. It needs the other Bs to use any one of them effectively. So when B-6 is prescribed for preventing miscarriage, doses of the whole B complex should be prescribed as well.

Roger Williams describes some of the pregnancy-preserving qualities of several other B vitamins in his useful little paperback *Nutrition Against Disease.* Pantothenic acid, for example, prevents fetal resorption. Rogers is credited with identifying and synthesizing this B vitamin. He describes a

French experiment in which female rats were given a diet deficient in pantothenic acid, and then allowed to mate. They conceived, but soon thereafter all the fetuses disappeared within the body of the mother. Another group of rats was given a small dose of pantothenic acid. Over half of the fetuses were resorbed. In a third group, about half the usual dietary quantity of pantothenic acid resulted in about 95 percent normal births and only a few resorptions and a few deformed infant rats.

What's true for rats isn't always true for human beings, but the study does point out the significance of even one deficiency in an otherwise nutritious diet. Williams comments that human milk is especially rich in pantothenic acid, and human muscle tissue contains about twice the amount found in other animals, so he suspects that we humans have a special need for an abundant supply of pantothenic acid. He writes, "I would be willing to give ten-to-one odds, that providing prospective human mothers with 50 milligrams of this vitamin per day would substantially decrease the number and severity of reproductive failures".[2]

Folic Acid

Folic acid is also extremely important for maintaining a normal pregnancy. Williams reports that in animals, folic acid deficiencies even as early as the first week after conception will cause fetal resorption and an end to the pregnancy. If the deficiency is produced artificially, beginning on the eleventh day after conception, 95 percent of the infant animals are born with deformities.

Vitamin C and Bioflavonoids

In most places in the body, the tiny blood vessels on the surface of organs normally just radiate outward in meandering patterns. If you had X-ray vision into the uterus during the first two weeks following ovulation, you would see an amazingly different design. Here, the blood vessels twist and turn round and round innumerable times, like tight springs, allowing a greatly increased volume of blood into the tissues lining the womb. This lining is the foundation for the nutrient-rich, spongy environment awaiting the fertilized egg.

In order for that egg to attach, burrow in, and continue its phenomenal development, this blood vessel–intensive lining must remain strong and resilient. Should the blood vessels break and discharge their contents, a woman would experience spotting between her periods. If too many vessels break, the lining's integrity is ruined and the egg cannot find a permanent home. The placenta sloughs off and the pregnancy is terminated in a spontaneous abortion. Enter vitamin C and bioflavonoids, a great team for increasing the strength of these unique tiny blood vessel walls.

In a study done at Cornell University over 30 years ago, 100 pregnant women with histories of spontaneous abortion took large doses of this dynamic combination of bioflavonoids and C, and 91 carried their babies to full term. Fortunately, bioflavonoids are readily available in fruits and vegetables—in the white inner rind of citrus fruits, and in green peppers, broccoli, parsley, potatoes, and cabbage. Supplements are inexpensive, and are widely available in ordinary pharmacies and markets, as well as health-food stores.

The most potent blood vessel–restoring bioflavonoid is called quercetin. It occurs naturally in quercitrin bark. This particular bioflavonoid is rather expensive, so most manufacturers do not include quercetin in their "mixed bioflavonoid" preparations. Buy a bioflavonoid mixture that specifically states on its label that it includes quercetin, or else buy this particular bioflavonoid separately, to make sure you are spending your money wisely.

Vitamin E (alpha tocopherol)

This is the vitamin most closely associated in the public mind with sexual function, although probably most people couldn't state why. In fact, research demonstrated that without this vitamin, male rats could not produce healthy sperm, or healthy, functioning testes. Also, fertilized eggs failed to implant in vitamin E–deficient female rats. There seems to be too little oxygen and nutritional support available in an E-starved placenta, and the fetus dies and is resorbed. When vitamin E was given to such females during the first week of pregnancy, the fetus was saved.

By 1975, there were over a dozen articles describing the use of alpha tocopherol to save a threatened pregnancy. Although the scientific community is still skeptical regarding the relationship of miscarriage to vitamin E deficiency in humans, this vitamin is known to have the following effects in the human body: reducing oxygen requirement of cells, preventing blood from seeping through blood vessel walls, bringing more blood into an area by dilating small blood vessels, and stimulating the body's creation of new routes for blood circulation. Common sense tells us that all of these functions are integral to the creation and maintenance of a viable placenta.

Vitamin E should be plentiful in a natural-foods diet with an emphasis on whole grains and seeds and nuts. But a woman who eats white rice and white-flour pastries and breads, and cooks with corn oil—which is deficient in alpha tocopherol, the biologically active form of the vitamin—instead of soy oil—which contains a mixture of tocopherols, including the alpha form—is asking for a vitamin E deficiency. We strongly suggest that women take up to 800 I.U. daily of vitamin E supplements if they have a history of spontaneous abortion and a diet deficient in whole grains, wheat germ, and soy oil.

This vitamin prevents miscarriage by allowing the egg to attach firmly to the uterine wall and a normal placenta to develop around it. Consequently, nutritional doctors advise their patients to take vitamin E supplements during the first four months of pregnancy, and then replace the E with calcium supplements. High doses of vitamin E prevent spontaneous abortion during those first few months; later, a prenatal multivitamin supplement plus conscious attention to a nutritious diet will provide enough vitamin E for the rest of the pregnancy.

So far we have discussed vitamin E for the woman, but miscarriage is often the man's doing, since it can be caused by a defective sperm, resulting in a defective fertilized egg. It is a good idea for your mate to begin vitamin E supplements, along with arginine and zinc, to help him create the healthiest, most active sperm he can. (If he has herpes, forget the arginine.) And don't wait until you want to become pregnant to initiate this program! Give your bodies time to heal and utilize these recommended supplements to their best advantage. Take vitamin E for several months, and then enjoy creating your healthy baby together.

Amino Acids

Amino acids are organic compounds that link together to form proteins. There are at least 21 different amino acids, and most of them are created within our own body. Eight of the amino acids that are essential to our health cannot be manufactured in our body. These must be obtained through our diet. Of these eight, tryptophan has a particular connection to miscarriage.

Nine pregnant rats were given a good diet that was deficient only in tryptophan. Eight were given the tryptophan as well. The eight reproduced normally, but none of the tryptophan-deficient rats produced any young. The researchers found out that after a few days of gestation, all the fetuses in the tryptophan-deficient females died and had been broken down by the female rats' bodies and eliminated.

Mother Nature doesn't go for singularities of any sort. She places multiple nutrients in multiple plants and animal tissues, to assure the continuation of her species. So, you won't find any animal flesh or eggs that contain every amino acid but tryptophan. Therefore, a tryptophan deficiency in a protein-adequate diet is impossible, unless the person's digestive tract refuses to absorb the proteins consumed. A newly pregnant woman, however, nauseated and lacking an appetite, might lower her food intake enough to suffer protein (and therefore tryptophan) deficiencies.

Daily Supplement Dose Advisory

Thyroid—prescribed by physician
Zinc—up to 50 mg of elemental zinc
Vitamin E—up to 400 I.U. d-alpha tocopherol
Vitamin C—up to 5 grams
Bioflavonoids—up to 1,000 mg total; up to 500 mg of quercetin
Folic acid—up to one gram
B complex—up to 100 mg
Vitamin B-6—up to 200 mg
Magnesium—up to 900 mg
Tryptophan—up to 1,000 mg

Chapter Ten:

Postpartum

In Brief—Postpartum

POSTPARTUM PSYCHOSIS (BABY BLUES)

Symptoms—Depression, insomnia, hallucinations, fear of harming baby, disorientation, crying spells, apprehension, withdrawal, manic behavior, lack of appetite, paranoia, mood swings.

Signs—Lower than normal B vitamin or DLPA levels in blood, low blood sugar.

Cause—Dietary deficiency or inefficient absorption of nutrients, coupled with stress.

Due to—Poor food choices or genetic defect; the physical and emotional stresses of new motherhood.

Solution—Improve diet; take supplements; eat more protein and more complex carbohydrates in small meals throughout day; seek help and support from friends, family, and possibly professional counselor; breast-feed.

Supplements—B complex, especially folic acid, thiamin, pantothenic acid, B-6 and B-12; calcium and magnesium; DL-phenylalanine, tryptophan, trace minerals, zinc.

POST CESAREAN

Symptoms—Generalized weakness; abdominal pain upon applying pressure to surgical site.

Signs—Abdominal scar.

Cause—Post surgical need for convalescence, recuperation.

Due to—Inability of obstetrician to deliver breech-position infant vaginally, fetal distress, maternal emergency, other medical reason.

Solution—Improve diet, eat more protein, take supplements, breast-feed.

Supplements—B complex, vitamin A, vitamin C, vitamin E both orally and topically on scar, calcium, magnesium, zinc, manganese.

EPISIOTOMY

Symptoms—Pain, itching.
Signs—Stitches, scar formation.
Cause—Surgical incision.
Due to—Impatience of obstetrician in facilitating delivery; obstetrician or midwife responding to a delivery occurring faster than perineal tissues able to stretch.
Solution—Improve diet, take supplements, sitzbaths, ice on stitches.
Supplements—Same as for cesarean, topical application of vitamins A and E, bromelain if tissues inflamed.

NURSING

Symptoms—Frequent breast-feeding.
Signs—Production of nearly a quart of milk a day.
Cause—Infant's appetite.
Due to—Infant's need for nourishment and immunological protection.
Solution—Careful choice of nourishing foods, frequent fluid intake, supplements, rest.
Supplements—Water; calcium; magnesium; zinc and trace minerals, especially selenium and manganese; vitamins A, C, and E; sunshine (vitamin D).

NOW, MORE THAN EVER, SUPPLEMENTS

You need nutritional supplements now just as much if not more than during pregnancy. Before delivery, your body was busy creating the skeleton, brain, and tissues of the fetus. Your vitamin and mineral stores were taxed to their utmost to provide for the two of you. Unfortunately, many women don't realize that after delivery, you are still providing for the two of you.

First of all, your body is depleted from the previous nine months' work creating the child within. If you took birth control pills until just before conception, you will be especially depleted in folic acid, vitamin C, vitamin B-12 and vitamin B-6, among other nutrients.

Second, your body is creating over a quart a day of the absolutely perfect sustenance for your baby. We will have more to say on the benefits of nursing later. It takes enormous energy to create that perfect infant formula within your body. You have probably already discovered that after you nurse you may feel like dozing along with your contented baby. Nursing not only requires energy—it also draws on your nutrient stores. If you have deficiencies in some vitamins and minerals, your milk can't provide what your baby needs for optimum mental and physical growth.

Third, your body needs nutrients to heal, whether it is from the major surgery of a cesarean, the minor surgery of an episiotomy, or just the basic stress and stretch of a normal delivery.

Fourth, if you want to avoid the postpartum blues, you must satisfy your body's need for the B vitamins and certain minerals.

BEATING THE BLUES

Postpartum depression runs the gamut from mild unhappiness to profound despair, from a sense of being overwhelmed to dark paranoia, wild hallucinations, and, in the worst cases, murder of the infant.

Possibly as many as 50 percent of new mothers experience some degree of the "baby blues." It is, after all, a rare new mother who doesn't feel as though she is sleepwalking after the first week of nighttime feedings and daytime caretaking, who isn't awestruck and frightened by the responsibility for the new life in her arms.

These universal aspects of new motherhood are frequently blamed for the common experience of postpartum depression. The fact that all mothers do not experience depression is explained away by the convenient excuse that those who suffer postpartum depression had a previously existing psychosis that was brought to the surface by the stress of giving birth and caring for a newborn. This diagnosis and explanation represents the grossest ignorance on the part of the physician and is a terrible, sometimes tragic disservice to the patient.

To illustrate more clearly what we mean, let's compare the symptoms of postpartum psychosis with those of common nutritional deficiencies.

SYMPTOMS OF POSTPARTUM
DEPRESSION
Depression
Insomnia
Hallucinations
Fear of harming baby
Disorientation
Crying spells
Apprehension
Withdrawal
Manic behavior
Lack of appetite
Paranoia
Mood swings

SYMPTOMS OF VITAMIN B-6
DEFICIENCY
Depression
Fatigue
Irritability
Convulsions

SYMPTOMS OF VITAMIN B-12
DEFICIENCY
Depression
Fatigue
Irritability
Mood swings
Forgetfulness
Indigestion
Crying spells

SYMPTOMS OF TRYPTOPHAN
DEFICIENCY
Depression
Insomnia

SYMPTOMS OF
PHENYLALANINE (DLPA)
DEFICIENCY
Depression

SYMPTOMS OF FOLIC ACID DEFICIENCY
Disorientation
Hallucinations
Fear of harming baby
Tremors
Irritability
Seizures followed by delirium

SYMPTOMS OF CALCIUM/MAGNESIUM DEFICIENCY
Depression
Insomnia
Fatigue
Apathy

SYMPTOMS OF HYPOGLYCEMIA
Apprehension
Anxiety
Crying spells
Apathy
Depression

SYMPTOMS OF THIAMIN (B-1) DEFICIENCY
Fatigue

Insomnia
Confusion
Emotional instability
Apathy
Numbness or burning sensation in hands or feet
Indigestion
Irritability
Depression
Fear of impending disaster

SYMPTOMS OF FOOD ALLERGY
Mood swings
Crying spells
Bizarre behavior
Compulsive behavior
Violent feelings
Irritability
Depression

SYMPTOMS OF PANTOTHENIC ACID DEFICIENCY
Loss of appetite
Indigestion
Abdominal pain
Burning sensation in feet
Cramping pain in hands or feet

It is clear that many of the symptoms associated with the so-called postpartum "psychosis" are quite possibly symptoms of severe nutritional deficiencies.

Two of the nutrients cited in our list of symptoms, tryptophan and phenylalanine, are amino acids. Both amino acids are components of all proteins, and tryptophan has been found to be a useful antidepressant when given alone in small doses.

Phenylalanine has been proved in a number of studies to eliminate depression in a majority of patients tested. Patients who were not postpartum but were hospitalized with severe depression, agitation, anxiety, sleep disturbance, and mental sluggishness were given a wide range of doses, from 75 mg a day to as high as 12 grams a day, without toxic side effects (except a transitory headache that disappeared within 24 hours), and with good results.[1] Tryptophan or phenylalanine are good alternatives to try when laboratory tests indicate no deficiency of B vitamins, minerals, or other nutrients.

Pregnancy, Dr. Carl Pfeiffer points out, requires increased zinc to provide for the proper growth and development of the fetus. He claims that almost "the whole human population is borderline-deficient in zinc." He also points out an interesting phenomenon: A male fetus will take up more zinc than a female fetus. Postpartum psychosis is more severe after the birth of a son![2]

In the past, home plumbing was composed of galvanized, zinc-lined pipes. Acidic water leached out the zinc, providing users with supplementary zinc, a much-needed mineral often deficient in diets relying heavily on processed, packaged, foods. Today, however, homes are more likely to contain copper-lined pipes, causing the average adult to ingest twice as much copper per day as is needed for health. Worse, copper and zinc are antagonists, so the more copper you ingest, the lower your zinc level becomes.

By increasing your consumption of zinc-rich foods and, if needed, taking zinc supplements along with other trace minerals such as manganese and molybdenum, you can lower your copper levels. You may even cure a condition that looks like iron-deficiency anemia but is actually a symptom of excess copper. As the proportion of copper to molybdenum declines through the use of zinc plus manganese in a 20:1 ratio, an anemia that doesn't respond to iron supplementation may, happily, disappear.

On page 144 is a recipe for an unusually nutritious chicken soup that the Chinese have traditionally given to new mothers during their first month postpartum.

POSTCESAREAN

If you had a cesarean section, you need to heal from major surgery. The trauma of any surgery affects your nutritional status, since the body calls upon its nutrient reserves to react to the physical and emotional stress of the experience, to heal the wound, and to ward off infection.

Poor nutritional status has a profound impact on postoperative recovery. Nutritional deficiencies are all too common, and greatly increase the rate of postoperative infections and other complications, even death.

High amounts of protein are immediately needed by the postsurgical patient.[3] Other important postsurgical nutrients include minerals such as magnesium and zinc, as well as calcium and manganese. Zinc is one of the most important of all postsurgical nutrients, for zinc deficiency is one of the most clearly tested and proven reasons for poor wound healing. Adequate zinc is crucial for cells to reproduce and close any wound. While many of the other nutrients are necessary for healing, they don't seem to *speed* healing. But there is some indication that zinc supplements can actually speed wound healing rates.[4]

Vitamin C is another well-documented element in healing, because it helps form the collagen that ties together severed body tissues, helps new blood vessels to form at the wound site, and prevents hemorrhage. Vitamin C also detoxifies the body from the anesthetics and other drugs used in surgery. Research has indicated that vitamin C levels drop after surgical operations, so we encourage you to add vitamin C to your list of daily nutritional supplements in the weeks and months following your cesarean operation. We advise you to add bioflavonoids to your vitamin C regime, because they have been proved effective for healing wounds, preventing and treating infection, and preventing hemorrhage.

Vitamin A is always mentioned when the subject of wound healing comes up and is also useful for countering the suppression of the immune system

Chinese Postpartum Chicken and Rice Wine Soup

    1   whole fresh chicken, about 3–3½ lbs cut into small pieces
    ½   cup ginger, sliced into ⅛ inch thick pieces
  8–10 small black mushrooms, presoaked, destemmed, cleaned
    ½   cup peeled raw peanuts (soak off brown skin)
    6   red dates, presoaked
  1–1½ to 2 cups dried wood fungus (presoaked, scrubbed with salt, and
         the tough parts removed) (known as *mook yee*)
    1   cup rice wine (gin can substitute)
    2   quarts water
         salt to taste

Heat 2 tbsp. oil in deep pan.
Stir fry ginger slices in it.
Stir fry chicken pieces, mushrooms, and mook yee.
Add water and dates. Simmer 15–20 minutes.
Add peanuts and rice wine. Simmer 5–10 minutes.
Discard fat that floats to top of pan.
When ready to serve, warm for 15 minutes.
Salt to taste.
More rice wine can be added at serving time.
Keep soup in the refrigerator.

This chicken soup is often served to new mothers during their first
month postpartum as a nutritious food that is believed to stimulate
breast milk. Red dates and wood fungus are available in Chinese
markets or herb shops.

that frequently follows major surgery. Vitamin A can be applied directly to
the wound itself, and we encourage you to rub vitamin A on your scar. Since
oral vitamin A supplements can be toxic in large doses, we recommend
increasing your consumption of vitamin A in the form of beta carotene,
which isn't toxic even in large doses.[5]

Various B vitamins have a role to play in postoperative recuperation.
Thiamine (vitamin B-1) and pyridoxine (vitamin B-6) are important factors
in connective scar tissue formation. Pantothenic acid (vitamin B-5) has been
shown to relieve postoperative constipation that can be caused by an anes-
thesia-induced paralysis of the small intestine. The B vitamins are called the
B complex because they work as a team. We urge you to buy a good quality
B complex supplement, or take brewer's yeast powder or capsules every day,
to assure yourself of adequate amounts of all the B vitamins. You will be
doing your nervous system, your mental health, and your postsurgical healing a favor.

Vitamin E is frequently mentioned in the medical literature as a useful means of healing and minimizing scars, used alone or with vitamin A.[6] After a cesarean section you have a double scar: the internal scar on your uterus as well as the external one on your abdomen.

Vitamin E, like C, also helps new blood vessels form at the wound site, and helps prevent blood clots. In fact, its usefulness in keeping the blood flowing and preventing the formation of clots can work against the formation of collagen and the repair of wounds, so we suggest that you apply vitamin E liberally to your scar but go lightly on supplements.

EPISIOTOMY

The episiotomy is a surgical incision made through the skin and muscle of the perineum, which is the area between the vagina and the anus. Episiotomies and cesarean sections seem to be techniques practiced by obstetricians here in the United States. Midwives in America and obstetricians in other countries perform far fewer cesareans and episiotomies.[7]

The episiotomy is a wound, and it's in a *very* inconvenient spot, one that interferes with your relationship to your mate, and to your new child because of the itching, pain, and discomfort, which last for weeks. You certainly want that incision to heal fast! Read the discussion on healing after a cesarean section, which describes the nutrients proven to facilitate wound healing.

An additional nutrient you may want to take, especially if there is inflammation around your episiotomy, is bromelain. Bromelain is an extract from pineapple that reduces inflammation and encourages drainage of fluid around a wound without interfering with normal clotting mechanisms. Bromelain has no adverse side effects.

NURSING: NATURE'S BEST NOURISHMENT

We are going to describe the supplements that are needed by a nursing mother to create the most perfect source of nourishment for her child. First, however, we want to briefly discuss why nursing is so beneficial.

If you expect to stop breast-feeding because you want to rush back to work, fear losing your figure if you nurse for more than a few weeks; don't like the sensation of full breasts if you've always been flat-chested; or just want someone else to take over at three A.M., we suggest that you reconsider. Thirty years from now, none of these issues will matter, while the adult child who was breast-fed for a significant number of months will still be benefiting from that intimate source of nourishment. Here's why:

· Sudden Infant Death Syndrome is less common among breast-fed babies.
· Breast milk changes its content according to the physiological needs of the infant.[8] The first milk, called colostrum, is high in protein and antibodies. The composition of the milk changes as the baby grows and matures. In fact, a mother's body is so in tune with the needs of her newborn that milk produced by mothers of premature babies is significantly different from milk produced by mothers of full-term babies.
· The longer an infant is breast-fed, the lower the adult cholesterol level will be.

- Breast-fed infants develop less atherosclerosis as adults (a clogging of the arteries and veins) than those who are bottle-fed.[9] In fact, some commercial baby formulas contain coconut oil, which is a 70 percent saturated fatty acid, often associated with premature hardening of the arteries.
- The iron content of breast milk, though quantitatively low, is absorbed far better than the iron in cow's milk, protecting the infant from anemia.
- The zinc content of breast milk is lower than that of bottled milk, but is better absorbed than the zinc in formulas.[10]
- Breast milk contains antibodies and an enzyme that protects the infant's intestine from foreign, allergy-causing molecules until the infant's own body can begin producing the enzyme, at about six months of age. Thus, breast-fed babies have fewer food allergies than bottle-fed.[11]
- Cow's milk is the ideal food for infant cows. Calves double their birth weight in 50 days, have four stomachs, and manufacture the casein-curdling enzyme rennin, which is useful because cow's milk is 85 percent casein. Human infants take 100 days to double their weight, own one little stomach, and don't manufacture rennin, as human milk contains only 40 percent casein.
- The fat in cow's milk differs from that in human milk; it is poorly digested by the infant and can lead to diarrhea, dermatitis, and even failure to thrive.
- Human milk has 4,000 times the quantity of infection-fighting lysozymes as in cow's milk, protecting the infant from fungus and bacteria.
- Children who were breast-fed have healthier teeth and jaws, have fewer cavities and need less dental work.
- Children who were breast-fed have fewer (or no) ear infections.
- Breast-fed babies have about half the illness rate and one third the hospital admission rate of bottle-fed babies.
- Breast-fed children are more intelligent than bottle-fed children.[12] One contributing factor may be the presence of the polyunsaturated fatty acid DHA (docosahexaenoic acid) in breast milk and its absence in formulas. DHA is one of the most abundant lipids in the brain, and lipids compose 70 percent of the brain's solid gray matter.

The Kind of Diet the Nursing Mother Needs

Producing a quart of milk a day will stimulate your appetite. If you satisfy your desire to eat by consuming high-quality foods, you will help prevent deficiencies of nutrients, such as folic acid, that are all too frequently depleted in the nursing mother.

When you design your weekly menus, do take the time and the care to include a range of fresh vegetables, fruits, protein, grains, sea vegetables, seeds, and nuts. Go lightly on dairy products, which are high in fat and are allergenic for many people. Include alternative sources of calcium in your diet, such as sesame seeds, dark-green and leafy vegetables, tofu, and soup made with soup bones and a variety of vegetables, plus a dash of vinegar to draw out the minerals from the bones. And eat sardines and salmon with fish bones intact.

When time is short, and it always is for a mother, make double batches of spaghetti, vegetable soup, and casseroles, and freeze some for fast future meals. Snack on yogurt, whole-grain crackers, fruit, hard-boiled eggs, and cut-up vegetables (diced in large batches and left in water in the crisper section or in sealed plastic containers, for fast and easy grabbing during the day).

The kind of diet we recommend, emphasizing natural, unprocessed foods of a variety of colors, textures, and food families, offers you the best chance to give your child a good start in life, whether you stay with a supplement program or not.

The Breast Milk–Diet Connection

Certain nutrients in your milk are more directly connected to your diet than others. Vitamin A, riboflavin (vitamin B-2), biotin (a member of the B complex vitamins), folic acid, vitamin B-12, vitamin C, and fatty acids are among the most directly affected. Zinc, iron, fluoride, and vitamin D are also affected to a lesser extent. Protein, lactose (milk sugar), fat, and calcium don't seem to be as affected by your diet. However, proteins can pass into the milk and cause an allergic reaction in your baby. Also be aware that otherwise healthy foods may be the cause of your infant's digestive distress: garlic, onions, sharp spices (curry, cayenne pepper) cauliflower, cabbage, and other gas-forming or strong-tasting foods can flavor your milk with tummy-wrenching substances. If the baby is colicky or cries often, revise your diet.

While we're talking about diet, beware of "dieting" while you're nursing. All those pesticides, herbicides, organic solvents and other chemical abominations of modern life are being neatly and safely stored in your fat cells. If you mobilize your fat as part of a reducing program, these poisons come pouring out into your bloodstream and into your breast milk, too.

What a Nursing Mother Needs

A nursing mother's number-one need is water! Keep a full glass at your desk at work, near you at home, and on your bedside table. Remember, you are putting out a *quart* of extra liquid a day in your breast milk.

You might have heard about beer's being a stimulant for milk production and considered it an old wives' tale. In fact, beer stimulates prolactin secretion, which is the hormone responsible for initiating milk production. However, there are beers and there are beers. We don't recommend typical commercially produced American beers, except for the brands that do not use any of the 52 additives, colorings, and stabilizers allowed by the Department of Agriculture in American beer. Do you want your baby to be supping on calcium disodium ethylenediaminetetraacetate (EDTA), F.D.C. Blue No. 1, Red No. 40, or Yellow No. 5? If not, choose your beer carefully—one of the increasing number of additive-free American brands or a foreign brand. (One dollar and a stamped, self-addressed envelope sent to American Home-brewer's Association, Box 287, Boulder, Colorado 80306 will bring you the complete list of possible additives.)

Brewer's yeast is the substance that gives beer its nutritional wallop and is an excellent supplement for the nursing mother, providing a rich supply of the important B vitamin complex and minerals. The B vitamins are crucial for nervous system development. Babies born to mothers deficient in B-12, for example, can also develop permanent neurological damage. B-12 deficiency isn't common, but should it occur, the repercussions on the child are severe. B-12 deficiency has been associated with low thyroid levels; since home testing for low thyroid is easy and free, we recommend that you test yourself postpartum for thyroid function (see page 35). If your test indicates you are low, improve your diet with added B vitamin sources (brown rice, brewer's yeast) and a B-12 supplement, along with a trip to your obstetrician . for his or her diagnosis.

Protein is an important part of the nutritional benefits of breast milk, and is also important for the mother as her body heals and strengthens itself after giving birth. An excellent source of protein is cold-water fish such as sea bass, salmon, and halibut, which offers the added benefit of omega-3 fatty acids (docosahexaenoic acid, or DHA), one of the most abundant fatty acids in the brain and the retina of the eye. Scientists have studied the effect of supplementing a lactating woman's diet with fish oils. They surmise that since the child's nervous system is incompletely developed at birth, the addition of omega-3 polyunsaturated fatty acids to the mother's diet postpartum facilitates the movement of DHA into the baby's brain, and, it is assumed, helps the optimum development of the child's brain, eyes, and nervous system. We feel that a mother who eats several fish meals a week does not need to take fish oil supplements.

Calcium and magnesium supplements, in a 2:1 ratio of calcium to magnesium, are generally recommended for all women in order to prevent osteoporosis in later years. During lactation, calcium and magnesium are especially needed, since the mother's body load of the minerals is severely depleted by pregnancy and milk production. The Joint Food and Agricultural Organization/World Health Organization Expert Group on Calcium Requirements has set 1,200 mg a day as the recommended dose of calcium. That means you need to take 600 mg a day of magnesium.

There is some indication that selenium supplementation of a breast-feeding woman can improve the selenium level of her child. Selenium is an important cancer-preventing nutrient, if not taken to excess. Yeast-derived selenium, as low as 50 mcg per day; is the safest and most effective way of raising serum levels of the mineral in the infant. We recommend obtaining the selenium in a good quality multimineral formula which reduces the number of tablets you must take each day and provides you with the spectrum of trace elements essential for health which might be lacking in your diet.

Zinc is another mineral we recommend obtaining in a multimineral. It helps induce the flow of milk and heal your episiotomy or cesarean incisions, and is essential for the proper growth and development of your child. According to Dr. Carl C. Pfeiffer, zinc is nearly universally deficient in the human population, and so we encourage the lactating mother to eat a diet rich in zinc and also to take zinc in supplement form. Oysters are the very best source of this mineral. In general, seafood, including seaweed, is a good source of zinc. Try crumbling toasted nori sheets onto other foods and soups. Eggs, brewer's yeast, mushrooms, whole grains, dark-green and leafy vegetables, legumes, nuts, and seeds are other good sources of zinc. You're at special risk of zinc deficiency if you eat prepackaged and refined foods instead of nature's bounty. We recommend purchasing zinc picolinate or aspartate, which are especially absorbable forms of the mineral. Any woman's healthy diet will include essential fatty acids, and a nursing mother is no exception. See on page 80 our description of the importance to the body of adequate fatty acids, especially gamma linoleic and gamma linolenic acid (GLA). Your baby's health, as well as yours, needs GLA, which you can obtain from cold-pressed, unheated safflower oil, evening primrose oil, linseed oil, borage oil, or black currant oil.

We do not recommend vitamin D supplements, either for you or your infant. There is quite a bit of controversy over vitamin D supplementation of infants, especially breast-fed infants. Breast-feeding mothers and healthy infants in our country really do not need vitamin D supplementation. Take your child out into the sun for a walk every day. Sunlight on hands and face will provide you and your baby with adequate vitamin D. You may need vitamin D supplementation if it's the middle of a winter storm and the sun doesn't shine for weeks on end.

Iron supplements are often prescribed for pregnant and lactating women. However, supplemental iron is a common cause of constipation and intestinal discomfort. The most easily absorbed iron form we know is iron citrate. (See in Chapter 8 "The Supplements Useful in a Normal, Healthy Pregnancy.") Whenever you take iron, in whatever form you take it, be sure to take vitamin C or a source of dietary C (such as orange, tomato, or grapefruit juice) along with it, to improve its absorption from digestive system to bloodstream. Iron supplements can hinder the body's uptake of zinc, so if your health practitioner recommends iron supplements to you, avoid taking the iron together with your other minerals.

If you are taking iron supplements, you need for vitamin E increases. It is interesting to note that newborns, especially premature infants, have special needs for vitamin E. Supplemental vitamin E taken by breast-feeding mothers prevents and treats the hemolytic anemia that occurs in vitamin E–deficient premature infants. We feel that you can satisfy *your* body's need for vitamin E in a good quality multivitamin tablet. The same goes for your need for vitamin A and vitamin C.

Vitamin K prevents hemorrhage. Since it takes a few days for a newborn's intestinal flora to produce this vitamin, many states insist that newborns be given an injection of vitamin K soon after birth. It is, however, a prescription item, not something for you to continue to take yourself or give your infant. Your diet of green vegetables and other nutritious foods will provide adequate K for you and your infant once you get home.

As you design a nutrition program for yourself and your infant, bear in mind the different characteristics of water-soluble and fat-soluble vitamins. Vitamin B complex and vitamin C are water soluble, meaning they flow out your urine within a day and can't be stored by your body for the future. So they need to be constantly replenished by your food and supplement intake.

The water-soluble vitamins, when supplemented, readily increase their levels in your breast milk. So be sure you know what and how much you are taking as you embark on a supplement program.

In contrast, the fat-soluble vitamins, vitamins A, D, E, and K, are stored in the body by your fat cells and your liver. Over time, your diet affects the level of these vitamins in your breast milk, too, but not as quickly as with the B complex and C. Since fat-soluble vitamins accumulate from day to day, you can overdose on them if you continue to supplement at high levels for months at a time. We urge you to follow our recommendations for vitamins A and E, and not use any more than we or your health practitioner advise.

With a healthy diet, rich with the natural colors of the rainbow and the textures of life, with breast milk for the little one and added nutritional supplements for you, you are creating the very best possible daily diet program for your own mental and physical health—as well as for the optimum mental and physical development of your child.

Daily Supplement Dose Advisory—Postpartum

BABY BLUES

B complex—50 to 100 mg of the major B vitamins
Multimineral that includes zinc and manganese
Calcium—to 1,000 mg
Magnesium—to 800 mg
Amino Acids—
    DLPA—750 mg three times a day with meals
    Tryptophan—500 mg three times a day

CESAREAN

Multimineral that includes zinc and manganese
    calcium—1,000 mg
    magnesium—800 mg
    zinc—to 50 mg elemental zinc
    manganese—20 mg
B complex—50 to 100 mg of the major B vitamins
Vitamin A—10,000 I.U.
Vitamin C—5,000 mg
Vitamin E—800 I.U. and Alpha tocopherol; may also smear on scar.

EPISIOTOMY

same as for Cesarean
Bromelain—400 to 800 mg

NURSING

Protein—20 grams extra

Multiminerals, including—
    calcium—to 1,000 mg
    magnesium—to 800 mg
    zinc picolinate—to 50 mg elemental zinc
    selenium—to 300 mcg
    manganese—20 mg
    iron—at least 18 mg

Multivitamin, including—
    vitamin A—to 10,000 I.U.
    B complex—100 mg of the major B vitamins
    vitamin C—5,000 mg
    vitamin E—800 I.U.

Essential fatty acids—safflower oil (several teaspoons), or evening primrose oil (1,250 mg 3 times a day), or linseed oil (1,250 mg) or borage
oil (one capsule), or black currant oil (as directed on bottle).

Chapter Eleven:

Menopause

In Brief—Menopause

Symptoms—Hot flashes and sweating, then chills; painful intercourse; vaginal itching; irregular or absent menstrual periods; urinary incontinence; mood swings, insomnia, depression, muscle and bone aches, and bone fractures are sometimes associated with menopause.

Signs—Increased gonadotropin levels (FSH, LH), decreased estrogen and progesterone levels, atrophy of ovary; osteoporosis also occurs frequently after menopause.

Cause—Drop in estrogen and progesterone; greater bone demineralization than rebuilding; psychosocial factors of family, culture, self-esteem.

Due to—Biological clock of human female in context of male midlife crisis, youth-obsessed American culture, children leaving and parents more needy, negative picture portrayed by media of middle-age female, inadequate consumption of calcium and other minerals, inadequate weight-bearing exercise, nutrient-poor diet with excess fat and refined foods;

Solution—Take supplements, decrease meat consumption, increase consumption of calcium-rich and other mineral-rich foods, digestive enzymes, exercise out of doors, make philosophical shift in perspective on stage in life, take steps to enhance self-esteem, reduce stress, avoid hysterectomy and, especially, ovariectomy.

Supplements—For general maintenance: multiple vitamin, multiple mineral, herbs; to fight depression: DLPA, tryptophan, B complex, brewer's yeast, vitamin C, zinc; for osteoporosis: calcium, magnesium, manganese, vitamin B-6, B complex; for hot flashes: vitamin E, selenium, vitamin C, bioflavonoids, dong quai; for insomnia: tryptophan, magnesium, herbs; for vaginal dryness: vitamin E.

The most creative force in the world is the menopausal woman with zest.
—Margaret Mead

It's important to remember that menopause doesn't last for the rest of a woman's life, although when she is in the middle of it, she may feel that it will never end. Some women go through hot flashes and an emotional roller coaster for a year, some for two years, and some for several years or longer. Eventually, however, the body finds a new balance, and any symptoms of transition end. So patience is one remedy, since time is the fundamental natural cure for the symptoms of menopause. Another remedy is to give your body the best possible materials that it can use to minimize the stress caused by the physiological changes of menopause.

Many of the distressing symptoms of menopause are caused by the body's cutting back on hormone production, especially estrogen.

We are made of the same materials as the rest of nature, and elements found in us are also found in the plants and animals around us. That means that there are sources of estrogenlike substances in herbs, roots, and other forms of vegetation, which can help ease us through the transition as our own bodies get used to a new, lower level of hormones, without putting us at risk of endometrial cancer or other harmful side effects of estrogen replacement treatments. Some natural sources of herbal estrogenlike compounds are ginseng root, licorice root, alfalfa extract, cucumbers, black cohosh, Honduras sarsaparilla, false unicorn root, lady's slipper, elder, wild yam, and passion flower.

To use herbs, steep one tablespoon of the herb in a cup of boiling water for a half hour or so, allowing for the active ingredients to concentrate in the tea. You may also find menopause-related herbs available in capsule form, as an alternative to loose herbs.

Ginseng and licorice can, over time, affect the cardiovascular system, so people with high blood pressure should not be taking these particular herbs without medical supervision.

Irene Simpson, a naturopathic physician in Arlington, Washington, recommends ¼ teaspoon per day of alfalfa extract for relief of menopausal symptoms.[1]

Herbs are the original drugs, so don't make the mistake of thinking if it's natural, it's harmless. Any substance that influences your physiology enough to be effective isn't always harmless! Herbs and can affect different people in different ways, but generally they work more slowly than drugs. You'll have the best chance of success and safety if you consult an herbalist before embarking on anything beyond a superficial exploration of herbs for menopausal symptoms.

HOT FLASHES

No one knows for sure why hot flashes occur and why anywhere from 40 to 85 percent of women experience this distressing sensation during menopause. We would probably know a lot more about flashes if men experienced the menopause. But until the mid-1970's, few researchers bothered to investigate a phenomenon that was first described in detail in 1927. Even today, the medical literature simply relegates the problem to a defect of thermoregulation, which means the body's temperature control goes wild as the level of hormones changes.

According to one explanation, "Estrogen travels through the bloodstream to the hypothalamus at the base of the brain, which is responsible for the control of basic body functions such as temperature. The hypothalamus registers how much estrogen is present and responds by secreting a chemical called GNRH, or gonadotropin-releasing hormone. GNRH travels to the pituitary gland, located near the hypothalamus, to stimulate the release of FSH, follicle stimulating hormone, and LH, luteinizing hormone. LH is responsible for ovulation. FSH stimulates the follicles to produce more estrogen. Lack of estrogen to the hypothalamus alters its function, and hot flashes result."[2]

Another possibility is that the flashes result less from diminishing estrogen levels, and more from rising levels of luteinizing hormone (LH) and follicle stimulating hormone (FSH). In fact, during menopause, the pituitary gland does secrete FSH at a rate several times higher than in premenopausal days.[3]

Hot flashes are not life threatening and have no known effect on overall health. They are a self-limiting condition; although flashes may recur for more than two years in some cases, they eventually *will* disappear without treatment. There are, however, inexpensive and effective natural remedies for hot flashes, so if the flashes are severe and disrupt your life, why not try them?

When natural remedies for hot flashes are discussed, two supplements are mentioned again and again: vitamin E and selenium. The two seem to work well together to control the abnormal temperature regulation that causes the flush sensation. Vitamin E was suggested as a remedy for hot flashes 50 years ago by a Canadian gynecologist, Dr. Evan Shute. Dr. Shute, along with his brother, Wilfrid, popularized the use of vitamin E for treating and preventing cardiovascular disease, among other conditions. According to Shute, vitamin E can relieve menopausal hot flashes in a matter of a month.[4]

Begin with 400 I.U. of E daily. Some sources suggest mixed tocopherols rather than alpha tocopherols.[5] If the mixed don't work, try the alpha. Over several days, build up the dose to 800 I.U. daily. If that doesn't lessen the flashes, take as much as 1,200 I.U., but no more. If the flashes don't go away immediately, keep taking the higher dose; It may take up to four weeks for the uncomfortable symptoms to diminish. Once they do, cut back on the E to 400 I.U. per day as a maintenance dose if possible.

Vitamin E does much more for a woman during menopause than help regulate body temperature. It helps prevent cardiovascular disease, retard aging by means of its antioxidant effect, reduce headaches, improve circulation, and prevent and heal varicose veins and blood clots. Don't use high doses of vitamin E without a physician's approval if you are diabetic or suffer from hypertension or rheumatic heart disease.

Iron and vitamin E don't mix well. If you are taking an iron supplement, be sure to take it many hours apart from vitamin E. Also, since E is a fat-soluble vitamin, mineral oil will draw it from your body if you use mineral oil as a laxative. Instead, choose a gentle, herbal laxative such as one made of ground psyllium seed. Estrogen itself causes a vitamin E deficiency, so if you are taking even a small dose of estrogen, be sure to add vitamin E to your supplement arsenal.

Selenium works closely with vitamin E as a detoxifier and antioxidant, and therefore as a preventive against premature aging. The two substances also strengthen heart function and maintain the elasticity of body tissues.

Vitamin C and bioflavonoids strengthen capillary walls. Since flushing is caused by the dilation of those walls, both C and bioflavonoids can help to minimize the effect of the flushing. Bioflavonoids are one of the best kept secrets of hot flash remedies. It is now 32 years since E. W. Cheng published the results of his studies linking flavonoids with naturally occurring estrogens, and 21 years since C. A. B. Clemetson published his study showing that women suffering hot flashes had weak capillaries until they took bioflavonoids regularly. The flavonoids strengthened the capillaries, and thereby indirectly treated the hot flashes as well. Two years later, Dr. Charles J. Smith published his own study of 94 women using bioflavonoids.[6] He gave them each six tablets a day, each tablet containing bioflavonoids—150 mg hesperidin complex and 50 mg hesperidin methyl chalcone—and 200 mg ascorbic acid (vitamin C). Each patient received these tablets for one month, and then were unknowingly switched to a series of tablets containing calcium carbonate, salicylamide, a drug that reduces fevers, and an estrogen. The bioflavonoids were "markedly superior" to all other substances in the relief of hot flashes. There were two unpleasant side effects: the women noticed a slightly unpleasant odor to their perspiration, and their sweat stained their clothing more than usual. It appears that bioflavonoids have some estrogenlike effects on the body, thanks to their structural similarities.

Dong quai is a Chinese herb that has been dubbed "the female ginseng." In China it is practically always part of any herbal formula designed for women. It improves blood circulation, and its folic acid and vitamin B-12 prevent pernicious anemia. Dong quai is also a sedative and analgesic, and has many other medical uses, including helping eliminate hot flashes, though it does not contain any estrogenlike compounds.[7] Consult an acupuncturist-herbalist for appropriate advice before taking this useful herb.

Dr. Norma McCoy, a San Francisco State University psychologist, and Dr. Julian Davidson, a Stanford University physiologist, discovered that a consistent sex life helped reduce the severity of hot flashes. Regular sexual intercourse may protect women from rapid lowering of hormone levels (the speed of the drop in hormones is suspected as part of the cause of the flashes). Whatever the reason, the women who had more frequent and regular sexual activity had less trouble with hot flashes.[8]

Common sense dictates that a woman experiencing hot flashes would want to avoid foods and conditions that make her hot. Large meals, caffeine or alcohol, and excitation caused by anger, joy, or any strong emotion dilate our blood vessels and causes us to become warmer. Other warmers are marijuana, tobacco (cigarettes diminish hormone secretion from the ovaries), electric blankets, direct sunlight, and warm weather. Sudden outbreaks of sweating can be uncomfortable and inconvenient, but both the discomfort and inconvenience can be minimized by simple measures such as sleeping on a large bath towel and keeping a fresh nightgown handy, and standing in front of a fan or taking a lukewarm shower. Also, avoid all clothing containing synthetic fibers. Natural fibers, especially cotton, allow your skin to breathe and help your body regulate its temperature. Also, drink plenty of pure water, a good all-around remedy for maintaining physical well-being.

Stress speeds up many of our physiological systems and is a potent influence on menopausal distress. "Stress aggravates hot flashes," says Dr. David Velkoff, director of the Drake Institute for Behavioral Medicine in Santa Monica. He has found that women who use biofeedback training to gain control over their nervous system can reduce or eliminate their hot flashes.

INSOMNIA

Some menopausal women have difficulty falling asleep. If you are experiencing insomnia, resist the temptation to take a sleeping pill. Sleeping pills prevent a truly restful sleep and can be habit-forming. Instead, give your body the nutrients that will help you relax physiologically, and give your mind sensations that will calm you and send you off to sleep.

Sweet potatoes and oatmeal are good sources of complex carbohydrates, and milk and yogurt contain calcium, fat, and tryptophan. Any of these substances may help you relax and fall asleep. Why? Your blood sugar may be too low, and may need a boost. That's a job for your evening snack. Complex carbohydrates stick around being digested for a longer time than refined carbohydrates (white flour and sugary products) and keep your blood sugar on an even basis during that period. In fact, as blood moves from mind to stomach for the job of digestion, you may finally feel drowsy. It happens that these substances also allow the brain to utilize an amino acid called tryptophan.

Tryptophan, when chained together with other amino acids, forms proteins. Alone, it is used by the brain to create a neurotransmitter (messenger from nerve to nerve) called serotonin. Serotonin in turn is a "calming chemical." According to Dr. Judith Wurtman, a research scientist at M.I.T., serotonin reduces stress and tension, and can make you sleepy.[9]

If you eat protein, you won't be able to produce as much serotonin. When several amino acids present themselves to the brain at the same time, the brain chooses certain ones over others, and tryptophan is way down at the bottom of the preference list. That's why the best way of obtaining a good supply of mood-calming serotonin is by not eating protein, but by eating pure complex carbohydrates. We know that sounds backward, but there is a simple physiological explanation. Carbohydrates stimulate the release of insulin from the pancreas. Insulin, besides moving blood sugar out of the blood and into body cells, also helps move amino acids out of the bloodstream and into body cells—all except tryptophan. Tryptophan clings onto a large protein called albumin in the blood and doesn't budge until it reaches the brain. By that time a majority of the other amino acids have moved out of the blood, and the brain has no choice but to use the tryptophan available to it to manufacture serotonin. We chose sweet potatoes and oatmeal as examples of complex carbohydrates that will set off the chain of events that will result in your brain's being flooded with this sedating biochemical. Any others will work just as well, including tortillas, rice, pasta, or bread.

You can also take amino acids as supplements, which are available at health-food stores. Never eat food when you take an amino acid supplement, or you've wasted money on the supplement. The body won't be able to use the amino acid in the presence of food (especially protein).

Magnesium is another calming, relaxing agent.

When it comes to calming the mind, reading the most boring section of the paper is one way to drift off to sleep. Massage is another delightful way to relax. If you don't have anyone at home (including a child) who agrees to massage you with gentle, soft strokes, close your eyes and massage yourself.

Light, restful music is an ancient remedy for relaxing and turning the cares of the world out. Ask at your local music store for suggestions.

Herbs, as mentioned earlier, sometimes work as powerfully as drugs, since they were the original medicines. Many people don't realize how many commercially produced drugs are synthetic versions of chemical compounds already devised by Mother Nature. Check with an herbalist and in herb books before you take off into the wilds of herbal self-medication. Valerian and skull cap are two mild herbs for helping you into a restful sleep. Valerian happens to be good for migraine headaches and indigestion, as well.

Light exercise is relaxing. Or take up yoga, which stretches and tones muscles and eases the body into a pleasurable sense of tranquillity. You can buy a yoga videotape, audiotape, or book, or attend classes.

Meditation is another useful relaxation tool; it can help you make better use of your awake time, in addition to helping you fall asleep.

VAGINAL DRYNESS

As the body's store of estrogen diminishes, changes occur in the vagina, including dryness. Estrogen keeps the vaginal walls thick and moist. A lack of estrogen coupled with the friction of intercourse can make the walls dry, crack, and bleed. This is uncomfortable but doesn't have to persist indefinitely. There are alternatives to dangerous estrogen replacement therapy.

You can use vitamin E oil to lubricate your vagina and heal the dry tissues. Cut or prick the end of a capsule of vitamin E and squirt it onto your fingertips. Massage the oil into the inner sides of the vagina. Intercourse itself helps treat vaginal dryness, as loving, relaxed foreplay stimulates the release of secretions. If you have no partner, self-stimulation will serve a similar purpose.

Besides vitamin E, calendula cream will help heal your damaged tissues. Calendula (marigold) has long been esteemed by herbalists for its ability to heal injured skin. Look for calendula creams in health-food stores or homeopathic pharmacies. Homeopathic medications are diluted natural substances that stimulate the body's defense system and promote healing without dangerous side effects. You can contact Homeopathic Educational Services, 2124 Kittredge St., Berkeley, California 94704, (415) 547-2492, for referrals, homeopathic medicines, and information about the use of homeopathics.

Daily Supplement Dose Advisory—Menopause

GENERAL MAINTENANCE

Vitamin A—up to 15,000 I.U.
Vitamin E—800 I.U. mixed tocopherols
Vitamin C—up to 5,000 mg or bowel tolerance
B complex—50 to 100 mg of the major B vitamins
Zinc—50 mg
Or a multivitamin national brand from health-food store, not a drugstore
   house brand
and a multimineral containing trace minerals such as vanadium, manga-
   nese
Herbs (see page 153)—1 tablespoon in 1 cup boiling water
Digestive enzymes (betaine hydrochloride and pancreatic enzymes)—as
   directed on bottle

HOT FLASHES

vitamin E—up to 1,200 I.U.
selenium—up to 400 mcg
vitamin C—up to 5,000 mg or bowel tolerance
bioflavonoids—up to 2,000 mg
dong quai—as prescribed by herbalist or check label in health-food store

INSOMNIA

tryptophan—up to 3,000 mg
magnesium—800 to 1,000 mg
valerian (if tryptophan doesn't work)—1 tablespoon steeped in 1 cup
   boiled water

VAGINAL DRYNESS AND ATROPHY

vitamin E—up to 800 I.U.
calendula (see page 157)

DEPRESSION

DLPA—750 mg three times a day with meals
tryptophan—up to 4,000 mg in divided doses during the day
vitamin C—up to 5,000 mg or bowel tolerance
brewer's yeast—up to 2 tablespoons
B complex—50 to 100 mg of the major B vitamins
zinc (elemental)—50 mg

Chapter Twelve:
Osteoporosis

In Brief—Osteoporosis

Symptoms—Broken bones, back pain, decreasing height, rounding of upper back.

Signs—X-ray examination of bones reveals loss of mass.

Cause—Lack of manganese, magnesium, copper, or calcium.

Due to—Inadequate diet, lack of sunshine, inactivity, poor absorption of minerals.

Solution—Eat mineral-rich foods, less red meat, more digestive enzymes, exercise out of doors, take supplements.

Supplements—vitamins A and C; calcium (in order of preferred forms: hydroxyapatite, citrate, lactate, gluconate, carbonate); magnesium; manganese; zinc; copper; silica.

There has been so much publicity in recent years surrounding osteoporosis that some women may believe it is an inevitable condition of aging. Not so. The people of Africa, Asia, and parts of Latin America are not breaking wrists and hips in old age as we Americans are. In fact, a 1970 report disclosed that the Chinese in Hong Kong and the Bantus in Africa suffer less from osteoporosis than the people of Britain and Sweden, in spite of the greater consumption of dairy products in the Western European countries.

In spite of the ballyhoo in the press about old age, osteoporosis, and never outgrowing one's need for milk, it's time to look the truth in the eye and realize that osteoporosis is a life-style disease, not a deficiency of calcium or a consequence of a long life.

FACTORS IN BONE LOSS

If you are still in your teens or 20's, you are at the perfect age to start building up your skeleton so it will be less likely to develop fractures later on. By the

30's, unless you are taking steps to keep your bones firm, some bone loss is beginning to occur. If you are past your 40's, you can still stop further deterioration and help your bones to remineralize. A number of factors are statistically associated with bone loss.

· Being a thin, Caucasian woman over the age of 60, or related to someone who suffered from osteoporosis.
· Having your ovaries surgically removed, which eliminates the body's major source of estrogen; estrogen has been found to help keep calcium in the bones.
· Heavy coffee drinking (more than two cups a day). Caffeine stimulates calcium excretion, reducing the amount of calcium in the blood, and thus stimulates the parathyroid gland to secrete the hormone that draws calcium from bones to replace calcium that has been lost from the blood.
· Smoking doubles a person's risk of developing osteoporosis.
· Having taken tetracycline, which may be used by dermatologists as a treatment for adolescent acne. We feel that this may be an unnecessary treatment at best and dangerous at worst, since it increases the excretion of calcium into the urine just when adolescent girls should be building *up* their calcium stores to prevent later osteoporosis.
· Heavy consumption of protein, especially red meats, which have 20 times more phosphorus than calcium, thus imbalancing the calcium-phosphorus ratio (which is normally a little over 1:1). Red meats may also stimulate release of parathyroid hormone, which promotes calcium excretion.
· Heavy consumption of other phosphorus-rich foods, such as soda pop and cow's milk. High-phosphorus foods cause calcium to form insoluble biochemical complexes, leading to inadequate absorption of whatever calcium is consumed.
· Heavy consumption of foods containing oxalic acid, such as chard, rhubarb, spinach, beet leaves, and chocolate. There is some evidence, inconclusive so far, that oxalic acid may cause calcium malabsorption. Since the vegetables containing oxalic acid have other benefits, eat them now and then but don't overdo them.
· Excess consumption of whole grain breads and cereals. Inside the husk is a substance called phytate which binds calcium into insoluble calcium phytate, making the mineral unavailable for use.
· Use of aluminum cooking ware, aluminum-containing antacids, aluminum-containing baking soda, or aluminum-containing underarm deodorant. Aluminum leads to increased binding of phosphorus, excess excretion of calcium in the intestine, and inhibited intestinal absorption of fluoride, leading to bone loss). There is also some suspicion that aluminum is a factor in the development of Alzheimer's disease.[1]
· Lack of adequate stomach acid, a condition called hypochlorhydria. This can result from drinking fluids at the same time you eat a meal, eating too fast and chewing too little, or from an organic problem with the stomach's acid production.
· A high-fiber diet, perhaps because fiber speeds food through the intestinal tract. Nevertheless, we still advocate a high-fiber diet, since in the greater scheme of things fiber is important for a healthy, effective, and cancer-free intestine.

· Lack of the necessary thyroid and parathyroid hormones to regulate balance of calcium between the blood and the bones.
· Lack of adequate vitamin D to activate the thyroid and parathyroid hormones that control bone demineralization and remineralization.
· Lack of adequate vitamin C to create the collagenous fibers to which the calcium of bone is attached.
· Giving birth to several children with very little time between pregnancies. Building the fetal skeleton draws a great deal of calcium from the mother's system.
· Taking certain medications, including some antacids, antibiotics, antidepressants, barbiturates, and cholesterol-reducing agents, corticosteroids, diuretics, and laxatives, and undergoing chemotherapy.
· Undergoing long-term steroid therapy, including using acne medications and topical creams.
· Alcoholism. Osteoporosis may be due to the malnutrition that usually accompanies this addiction.
· Immobility and lack of weight-bearing exercise. If you swim, be sure to take a walk or do aerobics as well. If you are bedridden, work whatever muscles you can each day; you may want to get some advice on an exercise program from a physical therapist.

FACTORS IN BONE RETENTION

Here is a list of the factors that contribute to stronger bones. Some of them you may not have read about before:

· Having active, healthy ovaries producing normal amounts of estrogen.
· Estrogen replacement therapy. Women must be aware of the dangers of this treatment, including endometrial cancer, meaning cancer of the lining of the uterus. According to a bulletin from the National Institutes of Health in May 1986, estrogen replacement therapy increases endometrial cancer from 1 per 1,000 women to about 4 per 1,000 women. Estrogen may also increase the risk of thrombosis (blood clot formation). When the dosage of estrogen is reduced and supplemented with another female hormone, progesterone, the incidence of cancer can drop, but is not eliminated. Estrogen *can* reduce the loss of bone, but it doesn't restore bone mass that has already been lost. The consensus of the NIH Conference on osteoporosis was that "there is no good evidence that elderly women should be started on estrogen therapy to prevent osteoporosis." We recommend using nutritional treatments first.
· Being black. Darker-skinned people tend to have thicker bones than lighter-skinned people. Men, also, suffer less from osteoporosis, because although they, too, lose bone mass as they age, generally their bones are thicker to begin with than women's.
· Weight-bearing exercise, such as walking, tennis, rope jumping, basketball, dancing. Exercise has been proved to increase bone mass even in elderly women with fragile bones who started exercising, so this may be the most important self-care technique of all, especially around the time directly after menopause, when bone loss is the greatest. An hour of exercise a day, three

times a week, is the very least amount of time to devote to weight-bearing exercises.

· Vitamin D, which helps bone remineralize but is dangerous in excessive amounts. Sunshine stimulates vitamin D production in your skin, so if you exercise out-of-doors regularly, you should not need to take supplements of this vitamin. Exposure of your face and arms to sunshine for a few minutes a day, or for an hour three times a week, is enough. Be sure to expose your skin for a few minutes *before* applying suntan lotion.

· Unsaturated fats in the diet, such as soy or safflower oil, which have a lower melting point than saturated fats such as lard or Crisco. Since those with high melting points inhibit calcium absorption, the unsaturated fats are the useful ones to preserve calcium.

· Eating sprouted grain breads and cereals. Sprouting breaks the lock that the phytic acid in whole grains places on minerals such as calcium and phosphorus, and allows these minerals to be used by the body.[2]

· Adequate bile salts. These substances are created by the liver and stored in the gallbladder. When fatty foods enter the duodenum, the upper portion of the small intestine, the duodenum releases a hormone that stimulates the gallbladder to release bile into the duodenum. Bile salts and water create a solution that emulsifies fats and oils. Calcium is absorbed along with the fats and oils. If you have trouble digesting fatty foods, you may need to take a bit more calcium. You may also want to see a nutrition-oriented practitioner for some advice on improving your liver function.

· Adequate thyroid and parathyroid hormones, which regulate the deposition of calcium in the bone.

· Adequate vitamin C, which helps the bones to use the calcium that is available in blood and soft tissues.

· Vegetarian diets. Heavy meat consumption is believed to disturb the calcium-phosphorus ratio because of the meat's phosphorus content. There is evidence that vegetarians in their 70's have greater bone density than meat eaters in their 50's. One researcher concluded, "When older women who ate meat were compared to similar women who were vegetarians, it was found that, even though both diets contained similar amounts of calcium, the meat-eaters lost 35 percent of their bone mass between the ages of 50 and 89, and the vegetarians lost only 18 percent.[3]

· Adequate hydrochloric acid in the stomach, which can be supplemented with betaine hydrochloride tablets before a protein-containing or calcium-containing meal. Note that calcium, like all minerals, is best digested on an empty stomach, when stomach acid isn't diluted with other digestive enzymes.[4]

· Diets rich in calcium-containing foods and drinks. These include low-fat dairy products, sardines and salmon with bones, dark-green and leafy vegetables like collard, mustard greens, and broccoli, tahini (sesame butter), egg yolks, nuts, beans, molasses and tofu made with calcium sulfate, plus bottled mineral waters like Perrier, which contains 140 mg of calcium per liter). If you experience gas, cramping, and diarrhea after drinking milk on an empty stomach, you may be deficient in lactase, the enzyme that helps the body digest lactose (milk sugar). About 31 percent of Caucasians, 45 percent of Orientals and 65 percent of Blacks lack this enzyme. Asians, Eskimos, Native Americans, and South Americans also commonly have difficulty digesting milk products. If you have this problem, eat only dairy products that contain active cultures of Lactobacillus bulgaricus and/or Lactobacillus acidophilus, which predigest the milk lactose. Choose a calcium supplement other than calcium lactate.

· Adequate magnesium. Magnesium activates vitamin D, which is required for calcium assimilation. Adequate magnesium ensures that calcium in the bloodstream is able to move into the bones and teeth. Even marginal magnesium deficiency can lead to calcium being deposited in joints, arteries, muscles and kidneys instead. The proper ratio of magnesium to calcium in supplement form is controversial. Janet Zand, a Santa Monica naturopath, herbalist, and acupuncturist, gives women who tend to be constipated 2 parts magnesium to 1 part calcium; women who tend to have diarrhea receive 1 part magnesium to 2 parts calcium; and women who have neither constipation nor diarrhea receive 1 part of each. Whatever the ratio, magnesium clearly is an essential supplement in any antiosteoporosis regimen.[5]

· Manganese, which is used by the body to create an enzyme that protects bone from demineralization.

· Vitamins A and C. In low doses, both aid in absorption of calcium.

We have not included sodium fluoride on this list. Although fluoride is known to harden bones, it can produce undesirable effects as well, such as pain in the joints, nausea, eye damage and peptic ulcers. The National Institutes of Health is currently conducting a five-year double-blind study on the health effects of fluoride supplements for patients with osteoporosis.

HOW MUCH SUPPLEMENTATION?

Absorption of calcium is notoriously difficult. Elderly women with little or no stomach acid and other confounding factors may absorb as little as 20 percent of what they consume. The body, being a clever conservationist, however, will absorb calcium with greater efficiency if there is real need for the mineral. The RDA is 800 mg a day, but at least 1,000 mg of calcium a day is a good amount for most young women, more if they have digestion problems. For pregnant or lactating women, or women over 40 who have no digestive problems from too little stomach acid, 1,200 mg a day is adequate. If a woman is over 40 and has too little stomach acid, then we advise her to take up to 1,500 mg of calcium a day. In normal individuals with average working kidneys and intestines, 1,000 to 2,500 mg of calcium a day have proved safe.[6]

No matter what your age or stomach acid condition, a dose of magnesium should be taken that is 50 percent to 100 percent the mg of calcium. Take a multimineral pill to provide adequate trace minerals. Folic acid and vitamin B-6 have been found to play important roles in new bone formation as well. Folic acid reduces levels of homocysteine, which can harden the arteries and possibly cause osteoporosis. In one study done in Sweden, though none of the subjects was deficient in folic acid, a dose of 5 mg of folic acid significantly lowered homocysteine levels.

At Harvard Medical School, Dr. Kilmer McCulley discovered that vitamin

B-6 can convert homocysteine into a substance that can be excreted by the body. Therefore, both folic acid and B-6 have joined the list of essential supplements necessary to counter the ravages of old age.[7]

Danger of Excess

One of the consequences of consuming excessive amounts of calcium is internal bleeding. This unfortunate condition seems to result from upsetting the calcium-phosphorus balance, which normally should be 1:1. If you take twice as much calcium as phosphorus, you risk interfering with vitamin K metabolism. Since vitamin K's function is to assure coagulation of blood, internal bleeding may result.

People who have an unusual sensitivity to vitamin D can stimulate too much D activity in their skin, and the body will absorb too much calcium. This condition is quite unusual, compared to the far more common danger of inadequate calcium absorption. Federal surveys have shown that 85 percent of women over age 20 consume less than the RDA for calcium.

Calcium is the major component of kidney stones. If stone formation runs in your family, talk to a nutrition-oriented practitioner before you self-dose with calcium supplements.

Women whose parathyroid glands secrete too much of the hormone parathormone, a condition called hyperparathyroidism, draw too much calcium out of their bones and into the bloodstream. Hypercalcemia, the condition of having too much calcium in the bloodstream, has resulted from ulcer patients taking more than 2,500 mg of calcium a day by consuming large quantities of milk and calcium carbonate antacids in addition to the calcium in their diet. This was more common before doctors realized that milk was not so good for ulcers, and before patients realized that antacids, taken in excess, aggravate the very condition they are meant to ameliorate.

If you are downing more than 1,500 mg of calcium carbonate (eggshell calcium) a day, plus drinking milk because you heard that's a good source of calcium, plus upgrading your diet with lots of dark-green and leafy vegetables, plus downing antacids because the eggshell calcium supplement makes you feel queasy, you may be in danger of developing milk alkali syndrome, a condition of excessive calcium that is uncomfortable and serious. In addition, calcium can precipitate out of your bloodstream and into the muscles and soft tissues of your body, creating other painful problems. You are in danger of developing these conditions if you regularly consume over 4 grams of calcium a day.

You can avoid this problem by using calcium citrate or calcium hydroxyapatite and throwing away those antacids. If you have trouble digesting your food, see a nutritionally aware health provider who can advise you in solving your digestion problems. At the very least, use betaine hydrochloride tablets before a meal and pancreatic enzymes after a meal, and see if acidophilus capsules or charcoal capsules will help your intestine to function better.

All Forms of Calcium Are Not Equal

Which form of calcium should you use? Some people use dolomite, which is actually marble dust, because it contains magnesium as well as calcium. Not only is dolomite very difficult for the body to absorb, it may also contain undesirable levels of toxic ingredients such as metals. Dr. H. J. Roberts of West Palm Beach was looking for an explanation for the unexpectedly high concentrations of lead, arsenic, mercury, and aluminum in the hair of some of his patients. He found that some of these patients were taking dolomite. He had one brand analyzed and discovered dangerously high levels of toxic minerals and metals in the supplement. Needless to say, we don't recommend dolomite.

Bone meal is another potentially dangerous form of calcium, since the bodies of the animals from whose bones it came may have contained pesticides, toxic metals, and other harmful substances, owing to modern farming and feeding practices. However, a refined veal bone powder extract was given, with good results, to one group of postmenopausal women who already showed thinning of their bones. In this study, the women were also given vitamin D injections and 800 mg of calcium glutamate orally per day, as well as 8 grams of bone meal extract. The researchers found that the women's bone density had increased after 18 months.[8]

Calcium is available in a number of forms, including lactate, carbonate, gluconate, or citrate. A few companies are manufacturing calcium as hydroxyapatite, which is the form it actually takes inside the bones. This form is the best absorbed, but it is also the most expensive.

Second-best is calcium citrate, because it provides the acid environment that calcium loves to have around it when it moves from the intestine to the bloodstream on its way to the bones. A study using 12 healthy volunteers at Baylor College of Medicine in Houston, Texas, compared the absorbability of calcium gluconate and calcium citrate and found that calcium citrate was as well absorbed by subjects with the least amount of stomach acid as by subjects with greater amounts of acid. Gluconate, however, was not absorbed at all in the subjects with the least stomach acid.

There are many variables affecting the efficiency of calcium absorption and takeup in your body, and the jury is still out concerning ideal doses in specific cases. You must exercise your own judgment using broad guidelines. If you are young and haven't yet overtaxed your stomach acid with excesses of overeating, if you're taking calcium mostly to deposit the extra bone to prevent problems in the future, and if you're looking to five or six decades or more of daily consumption, you could use the cheaper forms of calcium available. On the other hand, if you are starting to think about bone preservation later in life and need to do everything you can to halt bone loss immediately and begin remineralizing what is left, then we recommend sticking with the citrate or hydroxyapatite forms.

The quantity of calcium in these forms is not identical. Calcium carbonate is 40 percent calcium. If you swallowed 100 mg of calcium carbonate, 40 mg would be calcium and 60 would be carbonate. So if the label says, "Calcium carbonate, 1,000 mg," you are actually getting only 400 mg of calcium. Calcium lactate is 18 percent calcium, calcium gluconate is 9 percent calcium, and calcium citrate is 22 percent calcium. Microcrystalline hydroxyapatite is 30 percent calcium. Of course, the lower the calcium content, the more tablets you must take to obtain the daily dose you desire.

Always look at the label and check up on how many milligrams of elemental calcium are in each tablet, which is how much calcium is actually available to your body. Some products may claim that their amino acid–chelated calcium contains 500 mg of calcium per tablet. Since chelated products are generally one part mineral to ten parts chelate, 500 mg calcium would imply a tablet weighing 5,000 mg, which is three times the size that a person can easily swallow. This company is making an unreasonable claim, and an analysis of the tablet would probably reveal that a good percentage of calcium carbonate was mixed with some small percent of chelating agent.

Whatever the form and dose, calcium is stored in bone during the day and released from the bones at night to provide for body requirements during a time of no dietary provision. Consequently, bedtime would be a good time to take your calcium tablets. By supplementing at night, you will help reduce removal of calcium from the skeleton.

You have it within your power to protect your skeleton and to control, and even reverse, the degeneration of osteoporosis safely and successfully. All it takes is a healthy diet rich in minerals from land and sea, supplements of minerals and the vitamins that aid their absorption, and regular weight-bearing exercise.

Daily Supplement Dose Advisory—Osteoporosis

YOU ARE:

	calcium	magnesium
young, with good digestion	1,000 mg	600 mg
young, with poor digestion	1,200 mg	800 mg
pregnant or lactating	1,200 mg	600 mg
over 40, with good digestion	1,200 mg	600 mg
over 40, with poor digestion	1,500 mg	800 mg

a multimineral that includes manganese, zinc, copper
Vitamin A—10,000 I.U.
Vitamin B-6—100 mg
B complex—100 mg
Vitamin C—1,000 mg
Betaine hydrochloride and pancreatic enzymes—as directed on bottle

Notes and Further Information

CHAPTER 1. BREASTS

For Further Information

- Cancer Control Society, 2043 North Berendo Street, Los Angeles, CA 90027, (213) 663-7801, an educational organization that sponsors yearly conferences exploring alternative cancer therapies. Books, tapes, and other materials on the successful use of alternative cancer cures sold via mail order or at their library-bookstore.
- The Cancer Resource Center, 5880 San Vicente Boulevard, #103, Los Angeles, CA 90019, attn: Robin Bentel, M.A., (213) 933-8457 or (213) 838-4888, or Jack Tropp, (213) 664-0714. Worldwide telephone and written referrals regarding viable alternative cancer therapies and the medical professionals supervising these treatments.
- Cancer Hotline:
  Call 800/4-C-A-N-C-E-R.
  For information and referrals to support networks and medical help. Ask them for the excellent sourcebook *The Breast Cancer Digest.*
- American Cancer Society:
  Look in your local phone book for an office near you. The ACS sponsors mastectomy and radiotherapy support groups.
- Ellen Waisman, health educator, The Breast Center, 14624 Sherman Way, Van Nuys, CA 91405, 818/787-9911. A good resource for information, referrals, and counseling.

Notes

1. Pierre R. Band *et al.,* "Treatment of Benign Breast Disease with Vitamin A," *Preventive Medicine* 13(1984), 549–554.
2. Mark Wenneker, *"Breast Lumps: Is Caffeine the Culprit?" Nutrition Action,* August 1980, 4.
3. Robert M. Giller, *Medical Makeover* (New York: William Morrow, 1986), 54.
4. G.N. Schrauzer *et al.,* "Selenium in the Blood of Japanese and American Women With and Without Breast Cancer and Fibrocystic Disease," *Japan Journal of Cancer Research,* 76(1985), 374–377.
5. Kedar N. Prasad, *Vitamins Against Cancer: Fact and Fiction* (Denver: Nutrition Publishing House, 1984), 14–15.

6. Ernst L. Wynder, ed., *The Book of Health* (New York: Franklin Watts, American Health Foundation, 1981), 56.
7. Marie V. Krause, R.D., and L. Kathleen Mahan, R.D., *Food Nutrition, and Diet Therapy* (Philadelphia: W. B. Saunders, 1984), 741.
8. Kedar N. Prasad, *Vitamins Against Cancer: Fact and Fiction* (Denver: Nutrition Publishing House, 1984), 39–40.
9. Ewan Cameron, F.R.C.S. (Glas.), "Vitamin C, Carnitine and Cancer, or 'My God, I Feel So Much Better, Doctor!' " in *1986: A Year in Nutritional Medicine;* Jeffrey Bland, Ph.D., ed. (New Canaan, CT: Keats, 1986), 118–120.
10. G. A. Colditz *et al., American Journal of Clinical Nutrition,* 41(1985), 32–36.
11. S. Seely, and D. F. Horrobin, "Diet and Breast Cancer: The Possible Connection with Sugar Consumption," *Medical Hypothesis,* 11:3(1983), 319–327.
12. Melvyn R. Werbach, *Nutritional Influences on Illness* (Tarzana, CA: Third Line Press, 1987), 103.
13. Anonymous, "Urban Area Drinking Water Held Under Increasing Threat," *Los Angeles Times* (August 5, 1986).
14. Diane F. Birt, "Update on the Effects of Vitamins A, C, and E and Selenium on Carcinogenesis," *Proceedings of the Society for Experimental Biology and Medicine* 183(1986), 311–320.

CHAPTER 2.   UTERUS AND OVARIES

Notes

1. C. E. Butterworth *et al.,* "Improvement in Cervical Dysplasia Associated with Folic Acid Therapy in Users of Oral Contraceptives," *American Journal of Clinical Nutrition,* 35(1982), 73–82.
2. Seymour Romney *et al.,* "Plasma Vitamin C and Uterine Cervical Dysplasia," *American Journal of Obstetrics and Gynecology,* 151:7(April 1, 1985), 976–980.
3. J. A. Wylie–Rosett *et al.,* "Influence of Vitamin A on Cervical Dysplasia and Carcinoma In Situ," *Nutrition and Cancer,* 6:1(1984), 49–57.
4. Anthony H. Labrum, "Psychological Factors in Gynecologic Cancer," *Primary Care,* 3:4(1976), 811–824.
5. Carlo La Vecchia *et al.,* "Nutrition and Diet in the Etiology of Endometrial Cancer," *Cancer,* 57(1986), 1248–1253.
6. W. Schreurs *et al.,* "The Influence of Radiotherapy and Chemotherapy on the Status of Cancer Patients," *International Journal of Vitamin Nutrition Results,* 55(1985), 425–432.
7. Broda D. Barnes and Lawrence Galton, *Hypothyroidism: The Unsuspected Illness* (New York: Harper & Row, 1976), 133.

CHAPTER 3.   VAGINA

For Further Information

· Herpes Resource Center (HELP) P.O. Box 13827, Research Triangle Park, NC 27709. This nonprofit national educational program of the American Social Health Association offers information and emotional support to people with genital herpes.

Call or write the Center's Palo Alto, California, office, for referrals to local chapters of HELP, and self-help support groups, and for educational materials, including a quarterly journal, audiotapes, and videotapes: 260 Sheridan Avenue, #307, Palo Alto, CA 94306, (415)328-7710. The Center also offers private telephone counseling, a stress-reduction tape, and subscriptions to its informative quarterly, *The Helper,* which costs $20 per year. The Center sends all information in plain envelopes.

· The Santa Cruz Women's Health Center, 250 Locust Street, Santa Cruz, CA 95060. The 1987 edition of their 28-page pamphlet on herpes can be ordered for $4. It includes nonprescription remedies and a bibliography.

· Dr. David Sacks, *The Truth About Herpes,* Seattle, Verdant Press, 1988. This book is recommended by infectious-diseases researcher Maryanne Dillon of UCLA as "the best book on the subject," which is also the opinion of the American Social Health Association/Herpes Resource Center. Order it directly from the publisher: Verdant Press, 3963 W. 23rd Avenue, Vancouver, British Columbia, Canada V65 1L1.

Notes

1. Edward C. Delaha and Vincent F. Garagusi, "Inhibition of Mycobacteria by Garlic Extract *(Allium sativum),*" *Antimicrobial Agents and Chemotherapy,* 27:4(April, 1985), 485–486.
2. John J. DiGiovanni and Harvey Blank, "Failure of Lysine in Frequently Occurring Herpes Simplex Infection," *Archives of Dermatology,* 120(January, 1984), 48–51.
3. D. J. Thein and W. C. Hurt, "Lysine as a Prophylactic Agent in the Treatment of Recurrent Herpes Simplex Labialis," *Oral Surgery,* 58(1984), 659–666.
4. G. Eby, "Use of Topical Zinc to Prevent Recurrent Herpes Simplex Infection: Review of Literature and Suggested Protocols," *Medical Hypothesis,* 17(1985), 157–165.

CHAPTER 4. URINARY TRACT
For Further Information

· Interstitial Cystitis Association
East Coast Office: P.O. Box 1553, Madison Square Station, New York, NY 10159, 212/983-7620
West Coast Office: P.O. Box 151323, San Diego, CA 92115, (no phone). Offers referrals to national self-help support networks, information, and a quarterly newsletter.

· Homeopathic Educational Services, 2124 Kittredge Street, Berkeley, CA 94704, (415)547-2492. Homeopathy books, tapes, remedies, and home study courses are available from the director Dana Ullman.

Notes

1. Trattler, Dr. Ross, *Better Health Through Natural Healing* (New York: McGraw-Hill, 1985), 196.

2. Anthony E. Sobota, "Inhibition of Bacterial Adherence by Cranberry Juice: Potential Use for the Treatment of Urinary Tract Infections," *Journal of Urology,* 13(1984), 1013.
3. Robert S. Goodhart and Maurice E. Shils, eds., *Modern Nutrition in Health and Disease* (Philadelphia: Lea & Febiger, 1980), 223.
4. Kathleen McAuliffe, "In Pain, Sleepless—and Ignored," *U.S. News and World Report* (Sept. 21, 1987), 79.

CHAPTER 5.   MENSTRUATION

For Further Information

· The PMS Self Help Center, 19925 Stevens Creek Blvd., Suite 104, Cupertino, CA 95014. Susan Lark, M.D., director, (800)227-3900, (800)632-2122 (California)
· PMS Access, P.O. Box 9326, Madison, WI 53715, (800)222-4767 Free general information on vitamin and other therapies. For $9.95 they'll send a doctor's referral list and other materials, including books.
· Women's Health Advisory Service, P.O. Box 31000, Phoenix, AZ 85030, (800) 365-CARE. Founded by Dr. Sandra Cabot, creator of PMT-ese formula for PMS supplementation. Call or write the Women's Health Advisory Service (WHAS) and, for a small fee, they will send you preprinted information on the subject of your interest.

Notes

1. Carl C. Pfeiffer, *Mental and Elemental Nutrients* (New Canaan, CT: Keats, 1975), 225.
2. Richard A. Kunin, *Mega-Nutrition for Women* (New York: New American Library, 1983), 240.
3. Fuchs, Nan Kathryn, *The Nutrition Detective* (Los Angeles: Tarcher, 1985), 121.
4. Broda O. Barnes and Lawrence Galton, *Hypothyroidism: The Unsuspected Illness* (New York: Harper and Row, 1976), 124.
5. *Ibid.,* 124.
6. Karl M. Pirke *et al.,* "The Influence of Dieting on the Menstrual Cycle of Healthy Young Women," *Journal of Clinical Endocrinology and Metabolism,* 60:6(June, 1985), 1174–1179.
7. James R. Dingfelder, "Primary Dysmenorrhea Treatment with Prostaglandin Inhibitors: a Review," *The American Journal of Obstetrics and Gynecology,* 140:8(August 15, 1981), 874–879.
8. Robert S. Goodhart and Maurice E. Shils, eds., *Modern Nutrition in Health and Disease* (Philadelphia: Lea & Febiger, 1980), 137.
9. Jeffrey Bland, ed., *1984–85 Yearbook of Nutritional Medicine* (New Canaan, CT: Keats, 1985), 26.
10. Ross Trattler, *Better Health Through Natural Healing* (New York: McGraw-Hill, 1985), 440.
11. Robert S. Goodhart and Maurice E. Shils, eds. *Modern Nutrition in Health and Disease* (Philadelphia: Lea & Febiger, 1980), 340.

12. Broda O. Barnes, M.D., and Lawrence Galton, *Hypothyroidism: The Unsuspected Illness,* (New York: Harper & Row, 1976), 121–124.
13. Dominick Bosco. *The People's Guide to Vitamins and Minerals from A to Zinc* (New York: Contemporary Books, 1980), 25–26.
14. R.C. Robbins, Ph.D. "On Bioflavonoids," *Executive Health,* 16:12 (September 1980), 1–6.
15. Carlton Fredericks, "Female Dysfunctions, Hormones, Cancer and Nutrition," *Let's Live* (January 1984), 14.

CHAPTER 6. CONTRACEPTION
Notes

1. Robert A. Hatcher *et al., Contraceptive Technology 1986–1987* (New York: Irvington Publishers, 1986), 137.
2. James L. Webb, "Nutritional Effects of Oral Contraceptive Use," *The Journal of Reproductive Health,* 25:4(October, 1980), 151.
3. Judith J. Wurtman, *Managing Your Mind and Mood Through Food* (New York: Rawson, 1986), 20.
4. Bosco, Dominick, *The People's Guide to Vitamins and Minerals from A to Zinc* (Contemporary Books, 1980) 65.
5. Kosin Amatayakul *et al.,* "Vitamin Metabolism and the Effects of Multivitamin Supplementation in Oral Contraceptive Users," *Contraception,* 30:2(August, 1984), 179–196.
6. Frances Sheridan Goulart, *Nutritional Self-Defense* (New York: Dodd, Mead, 1984), 220.
7. Wilfrid E. Shute, *Dr. Wilfrid Shute's Vitamin E Book* (New Canaan, CT: Keats, 1975), 98, 170.
8. Broda O. Barnes, M.D., and Lawrence Galton, *Hypothyroidism: The Unsuspected Illness* (New York: Harper & Row, 1976), 134.
9. M. K. Horwitt *et al.* "Relationship Between Levels of Blood Lipids, Vitamins C, A, and E, Serum Copper Compounds, and Urinary Excretions of Tryptophan Metabolites in Women Taking Oral Contraceptive Therapy," *The American Journal of Clinical Nutrition,* 28(April 1975), 403–412.

CHAPTER 7. INFERTILITY
For Further Information

· Resolve, Inc., 5 Water St., Arlington, MA 02174, (617) 643-2424. A national nonprofit organization offering counseling, referrals, and support groups to people with problems of infertility, and education and assistance to associated professionals.
· Infertility Research Foundation, Elaine Gordon, Ph.D., 1460 7th St. Suite 301, Santa Monica, CA 90401, (213) 454-0502. A resource for anyone dealing with the psychological or medical aspects of infertility, or just needing information on the problem of infertility.
· *VDT News,* P.O. Box 1799, Grand Central Station, New York, NY 10163. $87 per year for six bimonthly issues. *VDT News,* a bimonthly industry watchdog, reveals important scientific studies and legislation regarding nonionizing radiation.

- Technical Information Branch, National Institute for Occupational Safety and Health, 4676 Columbia Parkway, Cincinnati, OH 45226, (800) 35NIOSH. Disseminates information on known effects of environmental and workplace hazards, such as chemicals and radiation, on reproductive health. A technical advisor will take down your questions and send you information retrieved from their computer.
- 9 to 5, 614 Superior Ave., N.W., Cleveland OH 44113. The 9 to 5 National Association of Working Women has a VDT hotline—(800) 521-VDTS—and publishes *The Human Factor: 9 to 5's Consumer Guide to Word Processors.*

Notes

1. Rose E. Frisch, "Body Fat, Puberty and Fertility," *Biology Review,* 59(1984), 161–188.
2. Joel T. Hargrove, and Guy E. Abraham, "Effect of Vitamin B-6 on Infertility in Women with the Premenstrual Tension Syndrome," *Infertility,* 2:4(1979), 315–322.
3. D.W. Dawson, "Infertility and Folate Deficiency: Case Reports," *British Journal of Obstetrics and Gynaecology,* 89(1982), 678.
4. Sheldon C. Deal, *New Life Through Nutrition* (Tucson, AZ: New Life Publishing, 1974), 55.
5. Masao Igarashi, "Augmentative Effect of Ascorbic Acid Upon Induction of Human Ovulation in Clomiphene-ineffective Anovulatory Women," *International Journal of Fertility,* 22:3(1977), 168–173.

CHAPTER 8.   PREGNANCY
For Further Information

- WaterTest Corporation, 33 South Commercial Street, P.O. Box 6360, Manchester, NH 03108-6360, (800) 426-8378, ext. 16. This company will perform a test on a sample of your drinking water to determine whether it contains lead or other contaminants.
- Cesarean Prevention Movement, P.O. Box 152, Syracuse, NY 13210, (315) 424-1942. CPM's purpose is to lower the cesarean rate through education, to provide a forum for women and men to express thoughts about birth, and to provide a support network for women healing from past birth experiences and those preparing for future births. A quarterly tabloid, *The Clarion,* is included with membership. $20/yr.
- C-Sec, 22 Forest Rd., Framingham, MA 01701. A support group for women after cesareans.
- *Silent Knife: Cesarean Prevention and Vaginal Birth After Cesarean,* by Nancy Wainer Cohen and Lois J. Estner (South Hadley, MA: Bergin and Garvey, 1983), $14.95. The best book available on the psychological and physical realities of cesarean, how to prevent one, and what to do to prepare for a vaginal birth the next time.
- *How to Avoid a Cesarean Section,* by Christopher Norwood (New York: Simon and Schuster, 1984), $8.95. Norwood, a woman, offers a useful manual to help you do everything you can to have a natural childbirth.

Notes

1. Marie V. Krause and L. Kathleen Mahan, *Food, Nutrition and Diet Therapy*, (Philadelphia: W. B. Saunders, 1984), 241.
2. Betty Kamen and Si Kamen, *Total Nutrition During Pregnancy* (New Canaan, CT: Keats, 1986), 151–152.
3. Judy Folkenberg, "A Bright Side to Morning Sickness?" *American Health* (October 1986), 88.
4. Robert D. Reynolds *et al.*, "Analyzed Vitamin B-6 Intakes of Pregnant and Postpartum Lactating and Nonlactating Women," *Journal of the American Dietetic Association*, 84:11(November, 1984), 1339–1344.
5. Judith L. B. Roepke and Avanelle Kirksey, "Vitamin B-6 Nutriture During Pregnancy and Lactation: II. The Effect of Long-term Use of Oral Contraceptives," *The American Journal of Clinical Nutrition*, 32(November, 1979), 2257–2264.
6. Carl C. Pfeiffer, *Mental and Elemental Nutrients* (New Canaan, CT: Keats, 1975), 151–152.
7. Thomas H. Brewer, *Metabolic Toxemia of Late Pregnancy* (New Canaan, CT: Keats, 1982), 12.
8. Gail Sforza Brewer, ed., *The Pregnancy After 30 Workbook: A Program for Safe Childbearing No Matter What Your Age* (Emmaus, Pa.: Rodale Press, 1978), 37.
9. *Idem, What Every Pregnant Woman Should Know* (New York: Penguin, 1985), 26.
10. Ray Peat, "Rosacea, Rhynophym, Pterygium & Riboflavin & Varicose Veins," *Townsend Letter for Doctors*, 49 (July 1987), 8707.
11. Ross Trattler, *Better Health Through Natural Healing* (New York: McGraw-Hill, 1985), 410.
12. Ray Peat, *Nutrition for Women* (Blake College, 1983), 55.

CHAPTER 9. MISCARRIAGE

For Further Information

· S.H.A.R.E. (also called Resolve Through Sharing), (608) 785-0530, Ext. 3696, 1910 South Ave., La Crosse, WI 54601. A national self-help organization providing counseling, information, and comfort for people who have lost a child through any means (sudden infant death, miscarriage, disease, accident). Includes S.H.A.R.E. Plus groups, for parents-to-be who have previously lost a child (before the current pregnancy).
· National Sudden Infant Death Syndrome Foundation, (800) 221-SIDS, 8240 Professional Place, 2 Metro Plaza, #205, Landover, MD 20785.
· Heartfelt, (818) 308-8222. Another self-help counseling and information source for people who have lost an infant or child.

Notes

1. Judy Graham and Michel Odent, *The Z Factor* (London: Thorsons, 1986), 16.
2. Roger Williams, *Nutrition Against Disease* (New York: Bantam Books, 1971), 56–59.

CHAPTER 10. POSTPARTUM

For Further Information

· La Leche League International, 9616 Minneapolis Avenue, Franklin Park, IL 60131, (312)455-7730. A nonprofit organization offering information and personal encouragement to breast-feeding mothers. A network of 12,500 La Leche League leaders offer free phone advice and hold monthly meetings throughout the United States, Canada, and 42 other countries. Bimonthly journal, books, and information sheets are available. Price list sent on request.

Notes

1. H. Beckmann *et al.*, "DL-Phenylalanine in Depressed Patients: An Open Study," *Journal of Neural Transmission,* 41(1977) 123–134.
2. Carl C. Pfeiffer, *Mental and Elemental Nutrients* (New Canaan, CT: Keats, 1975), 318.
3. John D. Kirschmann and Lavon J. Dunne, *Nutrition Almanac* (New York: McGraw-Hill, 1984), 116.
4. David R. Harris, "Healing of the Surgical Wound, II. Factors Influencing Repair and Regeneration," *Journal of the American Academy of Dermatology,* 1:3(September, 1979), 209–210.
5. Thomas K. Hunt, "Vitamin A and Wound Healing," *Journal of the American Academy of Dermatology,* 15:4, part 2 (October 1986), 817–821.
6. William B. Riley, Jr., "Wound Healing," *American Family Physician,* 24:5(November, 1981), 111.
7. Gail Sforza Brewer, *The Pregnancy After 30 Workbook* (Emmaus, PA: Rodale, 1978), 66.
8. Mihira V. Karra *et al.* "Changes in Specific Nutrients in Breast Milk During Extended Lactation," *The American Journal of Clinical Nutrition,* 43 (April 1986), 495–503.
9. G. R. Osborn, "Relationship of Hypotension and Infant Feeding to Etiology of Coronary Disease," *Collections of the International Research of Science,* 169(1968), 193.
10. Clare E. Casey *et al.* "Availability of Zinc: Loading Tests with Human Milk, Cow's Milk, and Infant Formulas," *Pediatrics,* 68:3 (September 1981), 394–396.
11. Mike Samuels and Nancy Samuels, *The Well Pregnancy Book* (New York: Summit Books, 1986), 182–183.
12. B. Rodgers, "Feeding in Infancy and Later Ability and Attainment: A Longitudinal Study," *Developmental Medicine and Child Neurology,* 20(1978), 421.

CHAPTER 11. MENOPAUSE

Notes

1. Irene Simpson, "Addressing the Concerns of Peri-Menopausal Women," *Townsend* (Washington) *Letter for Doctors* (April 1986), 89.
2. Stanford University Medical Center News Bureau, *Stanford Medicine* (Oct. 23, 1985).

3. Janet MacArthur, "The Contemporary Menopause," *Primary Care,* 8:1(March, 1981), 141–164.
4. Jack Joseph Challem and Renate Lewin, "Menopause: Natural Remedies for a Natural Event," *Let's LIVE* (November, 1981), 109.
5. Earl Mindell, *Earl Mindell's Vitamin Bible* (New York: Warner, 1985), 62.
6. Charles J. Smith, "Non-Hormonal Control of Vaso-Motor Flushing in Menopausal Patients," *Chicago Medicine,* 67:5(March 7, 1964), 193–95.
7. Him-che Yeung, *Handbook of Chinese Herbs and Formulas,* Vol. I. 177.
8. Stanford University Medical Center News Bureau, *Stanford Medicine* (October 23, 1985).
9. Judith J. Wurtman, *Managing Your Mind and Mood Through Food* (New York: Rawson, 1986), 62.

CHAPTER 12. OSTEOPOROSIS

Notes

1. Herta Spencer and Lois Kramer, "Osteoporosis: Calcium, Fluoride, and Aluminum Interactions," *Journal of the American College of Nutrition,* 4(1985), 121–128.
2. Anni Airola Lines, *Vitamins and Minerals: The Health Connection* (Phoenix, AZ: Health Plus Publishers, 1985), 81.
3. Robert Mendelsohn, "Osteoporosis and Calcium," *The People's Doctor Newsletter* 9, 4–6.
4. Roger J. Williams, *You Are Extraordinary* (New York: Pyramid, 1971), 305.
5. Nachman Brautbar and Helen E. Gruber, "Magnesium and Bone Disease," *Nephron,* 44(1986), 1–7.
6. Sara Benum, "The Experst Talk About Calcium," *Complementary Medicine,* 1:5(May/June, 1986), 9.
7. William Campbell Douglass, "Death, Taxes and Osteoporosis," *Health Freedom News* (April 1987), 19.
8. O. Epstein and S. Sherlock, "Vitamin D, Hydroxyapatite, and Calcium Gluconate Treatment of Cortical Bone Thinning," *American Journal of Clinical Nutrition,* 36(1982), 426.

ORGANIZATIONS THAT CAN REFER YOU TO NUTRITION-MINDED PHYSICIANS

American College of Advancement in Medicine
714/583-7666
23121 Verdugo Drive #204
Laguna Hills, California 92653
This group is especially focused on chelation therapy, but those physicians who do chelation are, themselves, knowledgeable about nutrition.

American Association of Orthomolecular Medicine
900 N. Federal Highway, Suite 330
Boca Raton, Florida 33432
800/847-3802
Orthomolecular physicians use nutrients as healing agents. AAOM is also associated with the Huxley Institute, a lay orthomolecular organization. This office has material on the use of nutrients for Candida, hypoglycemia, schizophrenia, depression, chemical dependencies, and learning and behavioral disabilities.

Price-Pottenger Nutrition Foundation
P.O. Box 2614
La Mesa, California 92041
619/582-4168
The Foundation is a source of information on the medical use of nutrition, as well as referrals.

Selected Bibliography

GENERAL HEALTH AND NUTRITION

Airola, Paavo. *Everywoman's Book*. Phoenix: Health Plus Publishers, 1979.

Bland, Dr. Jeffrey. *Assess Your Own Nutrient Status*. New Canaan, Connecticut: Keats, 1987. [Keats Publishing Company has dozens of health books and pamphlets, many written for the non-scientist, explaining individual nutrients as well as helping the individual to design an appropriate nutritional program. We recommend you send for their catalogue: 27 Pine Street, New Canaan, Connecticut 06840.]

Bland, Dr. Jeffrey. *Your Health Under Siege: Using Nutrition to Fight Back*. Lexington, Massachusetts: Stephen Greene, 1982.

Cummings, Stephen, and Dana Ullman. *Everybody's Guide to Homeopathic Medicine*. Los Angeles: Tarcher, 1984. Also, by Dana Ullman, *Homeopathy: Twenty-first Century Medicine*. Berkeley: North Atlantic, 1987.

Ferguson, Dr. Thomas. *The Smoker's Book of Health*. New York: G. P. Putnam's Sons, 1987.

Giller, Dr. Robert. *Medical Makeover*. New York: Warner Books, 1987.

Glassman, Judith. *Cancer Survivors*. New York: Dial Press, 1983.

Goldbeck, Nikki & David. *The Goldbecks' Guide to Good Food*. New York: New American Library, 1987.

Goodhart, Robert S., and Maurice E. Shils, eds. *Modern Nutrition in Health and Disease*. Philadelphia: Lea & Febiger, 1980.

Goulart, Frances Sheridan. *Nutritional Self-Defense: How to Use Nutrition to Counteract the Effects of Your Eight Worst Habits*. New York: Stein and Day, 1987.

Hausman, Patricia. *The Right Dose*. Emmaus, Pennsylvania: Rodale Press, 1987.

Hay, Louise. *You Can Heal Your Life*. Los Angeles: Hay House, 1984.

Kunin, Dr. Richard A. *Mega-Nutrition for Women*. New York: New American Library, 1983.

Lappé, Frances Moore. *Diet for a Small Planet*. New York: Ballantine Books, 1982.

Peshek, Dr. Robert J. *Searching for Health*. Riverside, California: Color Coded Charting and Filing Systems, 1982. [This book is written by a dentist who solved his own family's health problems by educating himself about nutrition and supplements, and doing research in his office laboratory on the effect of his treatments. His book has many unconventional and interesting applications of nutritional science to common female conditions. Order it from Color Coded Charting and Filing Systems, 7759 California Avenue, Riverside, California, 92504, (714)688-0800.]

Trattler, Dr. Ross. *Better Health Through Natural Healing.* New York: McGraw-Hill, 1985.

WOMAN'S LIFE CYCLE

Contraception

Chalker, Rebecca. *The Complete Cervical Cap Guide: Everything You Want to Know About This Safe, Effective, No-Mess, Time-Tested Birth Control Option.* New York: Harper & Row, 1987.

Trapani, Dr. Francis J. *Contraception Naturally!* Coopersburg, Pennsylvania: C. J. Frompovich Publications, 1984. Order from C. J. Frompovich Publications, RD 1, Chestnut Road, Coopersburg, Pennsylvania 18036.

Menopause

Greenwood, Dr. Sadja. *Menopause, Naturally.* San Francisco: Volcano Press, 1984.

Menstruation

Budoff, Dr. Penny Wise. *No More Menstrual Cramps and Other Good News.* New York: Warner Books, 1984.

Harrison, Dr. Michelle. *Self-Help for Premenstrual Syndrome.* New York: Random House, 1982.

Lark, Dr. Susan. *Dr. Susan Lark's Premenstrual Syndrome Self-Help Book.* Los Angeles: Forman, 1984.

Shreeve, Caroline. *The Premenstrual Syndrome.* San Bernardino: Borgo Press, 1986.

Osteoporosis

Notelovitz, Dr. Morris, and Marsha Ware. *Stand Tall! The Informed Woman's Guide to Preventing Osteoporosis.* New York: Bantam, 1985.

Postpartum

Kamen, Betty, and Si Kamen. *Total Nutrition for Breast-Feeding Mothers.* Boston: Little, Brown and Company, 1986.

La Leche League International. *The Womanly Art of Breastfeeding.* Franklin Park, Illinois: La Leche League, 1981. [For more information on the organization that supports and educates nursing mothers, look in the phone book for a local chapter of La Leche League, or contact headquarters at 9616 Minneapolis Avenue, Franklin Park, Illinois 60131, (312)455-7730.

Panuthos, Claudia. "The Psychological Effects of Cesarean Deliveries." *Mothering,* Winter 1983, No. 26, p. 61. Available as a reprint from *Mothering,* P.O. Box 1690, Santa Fe, New Mexico 87504, (505)984-8116.

Pregnancy

Brewer, Gail Sforza. *What Every Pregnant Woman Should Know.* New York: Penguin Books, 1985.

Goldbeck, Nikki. *As You Eat So Your Baby Grows.* Woodstock, New York: Ceres Press, 1986. Order from the publisher at P.O. Box 87, Woodstock, New York 12498.

Kamen, Betty, and Si Kamen. *Total Nutrition During Pregnancy.* New Canaan, Connecticut: Keats, 1981.

Mothering magazine, Box 1690, Santa Fe, New Mexico 87504, (505)984-8116.

State of California Department of Consumer Affairs. *Natural Remedies for Pregnancy Discomforts.* Available from Education Program Associates, 1 West Campbell Avenue, Building C, Campbell, California 95008, (408)374-1210.

Verny, Dr. Thomas. *The Secret Life of the Unborn Child.* New York: Dell, 1986.

NUTRITIONAL AND NATURAL HEALING

Brody, Jane. *Jane Brody's Good Food Book.* New York: Bantam, 1985.

Fuchs, Nan Kathryn. *The Nutrition Detective.* Los Angeles: Tarcher, 1985.

Null, Gary. *The Complete Guide to Health and Nutrition.* New York: Dell, 1986.

Padus, Emrika. *The Woman's Encyclopedia of Health and Natural Healing.* Emmaus, Pennsylvania: Rodale Press, 1984.

Peat, Ray. *Nutrition for Women.* Eugene, Oregon, Blake College. [Ray Peat is an irreverent, iconoclastic biologist who publishes *Ray Peat's Newsletter* to share his research and insights. Order the book or newsletter subscription from Blake College, 3977 Dillard Road, Eugene, Oregon 97405, (503)342-3004. Also available: *Progesterone in Orthomolecular Medicine.*]

Werbach, Dr. Melvyn R. *Nutritional Influences on Illness.* Tarzana, California: Third Line Press, 1987. Order from Third Line Press, 4751 Viviana Drive, Tarzana, California 91356, (818)996-0076.

Wright, Dr. Jonathan V. and Carol Baldwin. *Dr. Wright's Guide to Healing with Nutrition.* Emmaus, Pennsylvania: Rodale Press, 1984.

Wurtman, Judith J., Ph.D. *Managing Your Mind and Mood Through Food.* New York: Rawson Associates, 1986.

SPECIAL SUBJECTS

Cancer

Kushner, Rose. *Alternatives: New Developments in the War on Breast Cancer.* Cambridge, Massachusetts: Kensington Press, 1984.

Matthews-Simonton, Stephanie, O. Carl Simonton, and James L. Creighton. *Getting Well Again.* New York: Bantam, 1984.

Prasad, Kedar N. *Vitamins Against Cancer: Fact and Fiction.* Denver: Nutrition Publishing House, 1984. [Available from Dr. Prasad at 351 Fairfax, Denver, Colorado 80220. He has also published a technical medical text, *Vitamins, Nutrition and Cancer,* New York, S. Karger, 1984.]

Siegel, Bernie. *Love, Medicine and Miracles: Lessons Learned about Self-Healing from a Surgeon's Experience with Exceptional Patients.* New York: Harper & Row, 1988.

Herpes

Sacks, Dr. David. *The Truth About Herpes.* Seattle: Verdant Press, 1987. [This book is recommended by infectious-diseases researcher Maryanne Dillon of UCLA as "the best book on the subject," which is also the opinion of the American Social Health Association/Herpes Resource Center (ASHA/HRC). ASHA/HRC is a national self-help organization. The group provides other educational materials, such as a quarterly journal, *The Helper,* as well as audio- and videotapes on successfully managing herpes. For more information write to ASH/HRC, 260 Sheridan Avenue, #307, Palo Alto, California 94306, (415)328-7710.]

Yeast Infection

Crook, Dr. William. *The Yeast Connection.* New York: Random House, 1986.
De Schepper, Dr. Luc. *Candida: The Symptoms, the Causes, the Cure.* Self-published in 1986 by Dr. Luc De Schepper, 2901 Wilshire Boulevard, Suite 435, Santa Monica, California 90403, (213)828-4480.
Trowbridge, Dr. John Parks, and Dr. Morton Walker. *The Yeast Syndrome.* New York: Bantam, 1986.

Cystitis

Kilmartin, Angela. *Cystitis.* New York: Warner Books, 1984.
Shreeve, Caroline. *Cystitis.* Rochester, VT: Thorsons, 1987.

Hypothyroidism

Barnes, Dr. Broda and Lawrence Galton. *Hypothyroidism: The Unsuspected Illness.* New York: T. Y. Crowell, 1976.

Index